Acclaim for

W9-BSU-981

GETTING YOUR BRAIN AND BODY BACK

DISCARDED

"Riveting and compelling. At last, a book of hope for those who have been offered little in the past. Dr Berk's inspiring personal story combined with his empowering and evidence-based advice make this a must-read for those who have suffered catastrophic neurological injury."

—**Gary Gibbons, MD, PhD,** director of NIH National
Heart, Lung, and Blood Institute

"Dr. Berk is living proof that focused and purposeful mental effort can result in remarkable function, life satisfaction, and contribution to the world. His book provides expert and inspiring guidance for the many people who seek to overcome catastrophic injuries and get back to life."

—**Robert Califf, MD,** former commissioner of
US Food and Drug Administration (FDA)

"In his engaging and informative book, Dr. Berk puts the focus on patients and families, giving them the tools they need for successful rehabilitation."

—**Steven Kirshblum, MD,** senior medical officer at Kessler Institute
for Rehabilitation, chief medical officer at Kessler Foundation,
and chair of the Department of Physical Medicine and
Rehabilitation at Rutgers New Jersey Medical School

"In this important book, drawing both from his personal experience and the latest research, Dr. Berk shows us how to use the mind to restore the body. After thirty-six years of living with a spinal cord injury, finally words of wisdom can be put into practice."

—**Rob Tortorella,** executive chairman of
Corrosion Products & Equipment, Inc.

GETTING YOUR BRAIN AND BODY BACK

Everything You Need to Know
after Spinal Cord Injury, Stroke,
or Traumatic Brain Injury

Bradford C. Berk, MD, PhD
with **Martha W. Murphy**

Foreword by Eric Topol, MD

THE EXPERIMENT

NEW YORK

GETTING YOUR BRAIN AND BODY BACK: *Everything You Need to Know after Spinal Cord Injury, Stroke, or Traumatic Brain Injury*
Copyright © 2021 by Bradford C. Berk, MD, PhD
Foreword © 2021 by Eric Topol, MD

All rights reserved. Except for brief passages quoted in newspaper, magazine, radio, television, or online reviews, no portion of this book may be reproduced, distributed, or transmitted in any form or by any means, electronic or mechanical, including photocopying, recording, or information storage or retrieval system, without the prior written permission of the publisher.

The Experiment, LLC
220 East 23rd Street, Suite 600
New York, NY 10010-4658
theexperimentpublishing.com

This book contains the opinions and ideas of its author. It is intended to provide helpful and informative material on the subjects addressed in the book. It is sold with the understanding that the author and publisher are not engaged in rendering medical, health, or any other kind of personal professional services in the book. The author and publisher specifically disclaim all responsibility for any liability, loss, or risk—personal or otherwise—that is incurred as a consequence, directly or indirectly, of the use and application of any of the contents of this book.

THE EXPERIMENT and its colophon are registered trademarks of The Experiment, LLC. Many of the designations used by manufacturers and sellers to distinguish their products are claimed as trademarks. Where those designations appear in this book and The Experiment was aware of a trademark claim, the designations have been capitalized.

The Experiment's books are available at special discounts when purchased in bulk for premiums and sales promotions as well as for fund-raising or educational use. For details, contact us at info@theexperimentpublishing.com.

Library of Congress Cataloging-in-Publication Data

Names: Berk, Bradford C., author. | Murphy, Martha W., author.
Title: Getting your brain and body back : everything you need to know after
  spinal cord injury, stroke, or traumatic brain injury / Bradford C.
  Berk, MD, PhD with Martha W. Murphy ; foreword by Eric Topol, MD.
Description: New York : The Experiment, 2021. | Includes index.
Identifiers: LCCN 2021008686 (print) | LCCN 2021008687 (ebook) | ISBN
  9781615196951 (paperback) | ISBN 9781615196968 (ebook)
Subjects: LCSH: Movement disorders--Patients--Rehabilitation. | Mind and
  body therapies. | Spinal cord--Diseases. | Neuroplasticity.
Classification: LCC RC376.5 .B47 2021 (print) | LCC RC376.5 (ebook) | DDC
  616.8/3--dc23
LC record available at https://lccn.loc.gov/2021008686
LC ebook record available at https://lccn.loc.gov/2021008687

ISBN 978-1-61519-695-1
Ebook ISBN 978-1-61519-696-8

Cover and text design by Jack Dunnington
Author photograph by Matt Wittmeyer

Manufactured in the United States of America

First printing July 2021
10 9 8 7 6 5 4 3 2 1

To Coral, who carried me forward to a new life.

*To Mariah, Dave, and Sarah,
for their love and support.*

*To my many friends who unselfishly gave me
their compassion, support, and attention.*

*To the remarkable health care providers at
the University of Rochester Medical Center,
the Kessler Rehabilitation Institute, and
the Zhongshan Rehabilitation Hospital,
who kept me safe, taught me how to move,
and provided hope.*

Contents

PART 1
Your Recovery Begins in Your Head

PART 2
Functional Recovery, Health, and Wellness

Foreword

by Eric Topol, MD

BRAD BERK AND I were classmates at the University of Rochester School of Medicine and Dentistry. It didn't take long for me—maybe minutes—to know he was one of the smartest people I'd ever met. Our careers as cardiologists have crossed many times over the ensuing forty-five years we've known each other. We've both had major career changes, some due to opportunities and others due to necessity. But Brad's career has been nothing short of meteoric. Starting as chief of the cardiovascular division at Rochester in 1998, he became the chair of medicine in 2001 and assumed the role of CEO of the University of Rochester Medical Center in 2006.

But when Brad's life suddenly changed—after suffering a serious bicycle accident that left him a quadriplegic—that didn't hold him back.

He made a remarkable recovery and returned one year later to his role as CEO. After many accomplishments, he stepped down in 2015 to found the University of Rochester Neurorestoration Institute. Brad anticipated a dramatic change in neurorehabilitation, beyond the obvious personal meaning. He realized that devices would replace drugs for treatment of many neurological diseases and that these new technologies would promote neuroplasticity and recovery, changing millions of lives.

After his accident, Brad realized there was a paucity of information on the practical aspects of recovery from spinal cord injury, stroke, and traumatic brain injury. That's why this book he's written is so important. He refers to these three diseases as acute neurological injuries (ANI), due to their sudden onset and profound impact on daily life. Specifically, he's recognized the many features common in all ANIs, especially the psychological trauma. Finally, he foresaw the future advances in neurorehabilitation and the need for people to be prepared by keeping themselves as healthy as possible.

I empathize deeply with Brad, especially when it comes to the difficulties of finding proper resources to make decisions about your medical problems. In my most recent book, *Deep Medicine*, I tell the story of my own rehabilitation after a total knee replacement. I was born with a rare disease called osteochondritis dissecans. But the surgeon who replaced my knee didn't take my condition into account and prescribed the usual rehabilitation: aggressive movement of the knee to maintain full range of motion. Unfortunately, in my case, this caused reoccurrence of the cartilage and bone damage, leading to scar tissue. Thankfully, I was able to find someone with expertise in developing a rehab program that would work for me. As Brad emphasizes throughout this book, you and your family should be as educated as possible, so you can assemble a team that addresses your problems comprehensively and competently. This book will help you do just that.

A key feature of this book is the identification of similar problems among people who suffer an ANI. In particular, many people experience depression, frequently accompanied by anxiety. The modern-day poster children for ANI are individuals who experience a traumatic brain injury (TBI), such as our soldiers in Afghanistan and Iraq injured by explosive devices, and football players whose brains show evidence of a disease called chronic traumatic encephalopathy (CTE) and who often die by suicide as a result. Brad points out how important it is to treat these twin hurdles of depression and anxiety, so we don't lose valuable time for rehabilitation immediately after injury.

He also discusses two novel concepts regarding neurorehabilitation: continuous rehabilitation and the use of integrative medicine. The benefit of continuous rehabilitation is evidenced by Brad himself, who chronicles his slow-but-steady improvement in regaining many aspects of his prior life, including sports such as cycling and skiing, and daily physical therapy and exercise. Particularly interesting for me was his discussion of integrative medicine; he recommends incorporating several aspects of traditional Chinese medicine as complements to Western medicine.

While I found the whole book fascinating, the last chapter in part four was the most enjoyable, since my own three books all dealt with how novel technology influences medicine. This is an exciting time for neurorehabilitation, and Brad combines the best elements of the past with a carefully justified focus on future therapies.

While he and I were at the University of Rochester, we were taught the biopsychosocial model of medicine, which emphasizes the critical role of the environment and your mental health in determining illness. When Brad was CEO of URMC, he initiated a patient-and-family-centered care program that focused on compassion and attentiveness. Compassion is the natural feeling that people in health care bring to their patient interaction by showing that they care about them. Attentiveness is how we show compassion. Brad's book provides healthy amounts of both for patients, families, and providers. The promises of future devices that will enable people to walk—and eventually, to use their brains to control their paralyzed limbs—cannot be considered in isolation. The best practice of medicine remains an art, and Brad has painted an encouraging picture of present and future recovery.

It is an honor to write this foreword. Brad's book is essential for everyone who has experienced a spinal cord injury, stroke, or traumatic brain injury.

Eric Topol, MD
January 29, 2021

Eric Topol, MD, is the founder and director of the Scripps Translational Science Institute, a professor of molecular medicine, and executive vice president of Scripps Research. One of the top ten most cited researchers in medicine, Topol was elected to the National Academy of Medicine and has led many of the trials that have shaped contemporary treatment for heart disease. He lives in La Jolla, California.

Why I Know You Can
Get Back to Life

Y STORY BEGINS on May 30, 2009, when I took a bike ride that changed my life.

It was Memorial Day weekend, and my wife and I were at our vacation cottage on Canandaigua Lake, one of the Finger Lakes in upstate New York. Our three children, all adults with their own careers by then, had come to join us for the long weekend. It was a family tradition for us to gather at the lake house for holidays, summer vacations, and whenever we could get away. Being there, away from the demands of our jobs and daily routines, gave us the opportunity to just hang out together, enjoy leisurely meals, play games, and take walks and bike rides.

The Finger Lakes region, an area southeast of Rochester (where we lived and worked), is one of rolling hills and panoramic vistas of farms, forests, and lakes. It was my favorite place to cycle. I had always loved long-distance biking; at the lake, I began taking frequent 50-mile rides— and longer. It was such a perfect place for cycling that, during July and August, I would take Fridays off from my demanding work as CEO of the University of Rochester Medical Center (URMC), a large health care system with multiple hospitals, just to get in a six-hour, 100-mile ride during the day. The best part of the ride was the last four miles, which included a ride up a big hill to an area called The Bluffs. There was a breathtaking view from the top of the hill and an exhilarating ride down—tailor-made for an experienced cyclist.

The weather was beautiful, so on that Sunday afternoon, I decided to take a quick 20-mile ride before the barbecue we'd planned for that evening. Perched atop The Bluffs, sipping some water and taking in the scenery, I checked the road below me before getting back on the bike to head home. All clear.

I blasted down the hill, lost in the euphoria of the workout and the scenery. My muscle memory kicked in as I leaned the bike into the hair-pin curve of the road I had ridden a hundred times before.

I heard the car before I saw it, but I looked up just in time to find a large white station wagon taking up the entire road. I quickly realized I couldn't go around the car without flying over the guardrail and tumbling down a deep ravine. At thirty miles per hour, I couldn't slow down without hitting the car head-on and being thrown onto the windshield. So I tried a mountain-bike maneuver: I shifted my weight back and skidded the rear tire around to try to slide under the car.

As I gently squeezed the brakes and started the skid, I felt myself being thrown over the handlebars. I heard a loud crack and landed headfirst on the ground. I learned later that the skid caused my rear tire to blow, which made the bike wobble and nearly stop, sending me forward.

I noticed instantly that I couldn't move my legs or my left arm. When I tried pulling my right arm underneath me to push myself up, it too stopped moving. I could tell that my neck was broken. Even worse, I was panting, which meant my injury was probably above the fifth cervical vertebra—since that part of the spinal cord contains the nerves that control the diaphragm and breathing.

A man was walking toward me from the car. He looked down at me, surprised and concerned. I asked him to call 911 and to get my phone out of my bag so that I could call my family. He dialed and placed the phone next to my ear. When my son Dave answered the phone, I told him what had happened. "By the tone of your voice, Dad, I knew it was something really bad," he told me later, "We drove there terrified about what we would find."

They had every reason to be worried.

Within ten minutes of the 911 call, a police officer showed up and an ambulance arrived. I was loaded into the ambulance and driven to a large grassy field where an emergency medical helicopter waited. The entrance into the cargo bay was narrow and dark, claustrophobic. When the helicopter took off, the noise was deafening, and the darkness only heightened my fear and anxiety. But, surprisingly, I don't recall feeling any pain. I don't know if this was due to a loss of sensation or being in shock, but I was grateful for it at the time. Finally, the helicopter landed on the roof of URMC's major trauma facility, Strong Memorial

Hospital. I thought I was prepared for what would happen next, because I had experience taking care of soldiers with spinal cord injuries during my residency.

I wasn't.

No one is prepared for the life-changing event of spinal cord injury, stroke, or traumatic brain injury. In an instant, your world is turned upside down, and the future, if you can even picture one, looks terrifying.

The next twenty-four hours were a blur. I needed surgery to stabilize my spine with titanium rods and trusses. When I woke up, I was not surprised to be on a ventilator, but in my wildest dreams I could not have imagined how uncomfortable it would be. After surgery, I spent ten days in the ICU hooked up to the ventilator, unable to speak, move, or feel below my neck. I was a quadriplegic: I had paralysis of all four limbs.

I spent months in the hospital, first in intensive care and then in a rehabilitation hospital. I had to learn how to breathe again as I was weaned off the ventilator. I had to learn how to swallow again. I had to surrender my sense of modesty and allow others to help me use a toilet. When I was finally able to go "home" again, I had to move from a house I loved and had lived in for many years into an accessible townhouse.

My world had been turned upside down. And I know yours has too. Which is why I wrote this book, to give you all the information I wish I'd known at the time of my accident and beyond.

Like every person who has suffered an acute neurological injury (ANI), I was told that the first twelve months would reveal the limits of my neurological recovery, the *this is as good as it's gonna get for you* scenario. Thankfully, that depressing prediction proved to be untrue. My recovery continued long past the twelve-month mark; it continues to this day. If you've been told to believe that a similar limit exists for you, I hope this book will show you otherwise. Just as important, I hope it offers you and your family hope, compassion, pep talks, and understanding. After all, I'm a guy who's been there.

My spinal cord injury took me from the top of the world to the depths of despair. It was the most difficult experience I have ever faced. Today, I'm back on top of the world—a rewarding job, a rich family life, a happy marriage. I'm active in my community, and I'm an advocate at the local and state level for those with disabilities. Life is good. In many ways, I've become a better person—not *despite* my injury but because of it.

I'm also a better doctor. My spinal cord injury changed my view of the patient–physician relationship, the value of mind-body approaches to medicine, and the very meaning of life.

Having an ANI is one of the most serious challenges anyone will face. Ultimately, what I've learned is that each day offers opportunities for joy. I hope the information in this book will help you on your journey back to a meaningful life filled with love.

Brad Berk, MD, PhD
February 4, 2021

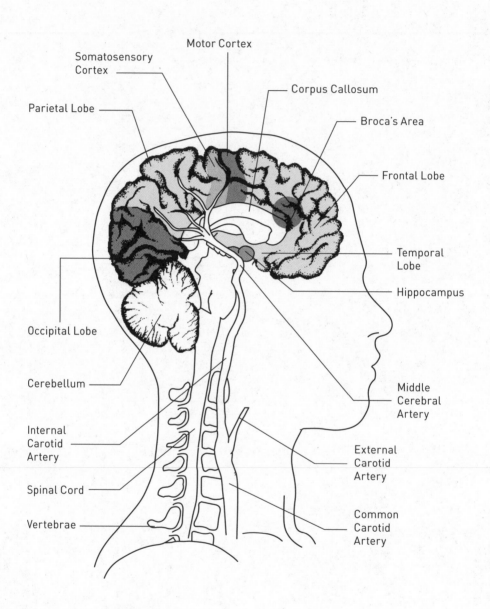

Motor Cortex

Somatosensory
Cortex

Corpus Callosum

Parietal Lobe

Broca's Area

Frontal Lobe

Temporal
Lobe

Hippocampus

Occipital Lobe

Middle
Cerebral
Artery

Cerebellum

Internal
Carotid
Artery

External
Carotid
Artery

Spinal Cord

Common
Carotid
Artery

Vertebrae

Figure 1: The brain and spinal cord

What Is An Acute Neurological Injury?

Explaining Spinal Cord Injury, Stroke, and Traumatic Brain Injury

You MAY WONDER WHY I wrote about three different neurological injuries, rather than about spinal cord injury (SCI) alone. If you've experienced an SCI, stroke, or traumatic brain injury (TBI), your injury is considered an acute neurological injury (ANI). These three conditions result in many of the same physical disabilities: paralysis and loss of sensation, of course, but also difficulty eating, sleeping, breathing, exercising, having a bowel movement, communicating (speaking, hearing, and understanding language), and performing many activities of daily living. They also share many psychological and mental health disorders: anxiety, depression, emotional lability, grief, and post-traumatic stress disorder (PTSD).

ANIs share many of the same therapies and treatments—during hospital care and outpatient rehabilitation—which is why the person next to you at physical therapy may be going through the same balance and walking exercises as you, even though you've had a stroke and she's had a TBI. Many of the medications are the same, and many assistive devices are useful for anyone with an ANI. Whether you've experienced a stroke, SCI, or TBI, you may find the advice given here to be helpful for your recovery. You'll also, of course, find advice for your particular ANI throughout.

To help you understand the physical aspects of the ANIs, here's a brief anatomy lesson (Figure 1). Dr. David Goldstein, chief of the Autonomic Medicine Section at the National Institute of Neurological Disorders and Stroke, describes the central nervous system as "like a Tootsie Roll pop. The brain is the candy. The spinal cord is the stick. The chewy chocolate center is the brainstem."[1] The brain consists of all tissues within your skull from the brainstem upward. It's divided into four lobes based on their overlying neurocranial bones. Counterclockwise, they are the frontal, parietal, occipital, and temporal lobes. In Figure 1, the temporal lobe was removed to expose the hippocampus (center of memory and learning), Broca's area (center of speech and language), and the corpus callosum (a large collection of nerves that connect the two halves of the brain). The cerebrum of the brain is the uppermost region of the central nervous system. With the cerebellum, it controls all voluntary actions of the human body. The cerebral cortex is the outer layer of nerves in the cerebrum and is the largest site of nerve connections, processing of information, and source of movement and activities. It plays a key role in thought, memory, language, and consciousness. The spinal cord begins where the bottom of the brain (the brainstem) exits the skull. The upper part of the spinal cord is the cervical region, with seven vertebrae. The brain receives blood and nutrition via the carotid arteries in the front and the vertebral arteries in the back (not shown).

The Three ANIs: Spinal Cord Injury, Stroke, and Traumatic Brain Injury

Spinal Cord Injury (SCI): SCI is damage to the spinal cord that causes immediate changes in function of the body at or below the site of injury. The extent of the injury is determined by the vertebrae of the spine, which are divided into four parts, each with its own number of bones. Just below the entrance to the brain are the cervical vertebrae (C1 to C7, Figure 2A), followed by the thoracic (T1 to T12), the lumbar (L1 to L5), and finally the sacral vertebrae (S1 to S5) at the bottom. Doctors "map" the spinal cord to the body by using sensation to identify regions of the skin, called dermatomes, that are supplied by nerves that exit the spinal cord at specific sites. For example, the thumb and forefinger are innervated by C6, while the nipples are innervated by T6 (Figure 2B). These sites are also where nerves that control muscle movement (motor neurons) exit the spinal cord, so that damage to C6 will paralyze the wrist flexors, triceps, and thumb and forefinger (Figure 2C). The higher the SCI (the closer to your brain), the more severe the motor and sensory deficits. Above T1 to C7, you will be a tetraplegic, with weakness in both your legs and hands (Figures 2B and 2C). Long-term outcomes range widely, from full recovery to permanent tetraplegia (also called quadriplegia, meaning paralysis

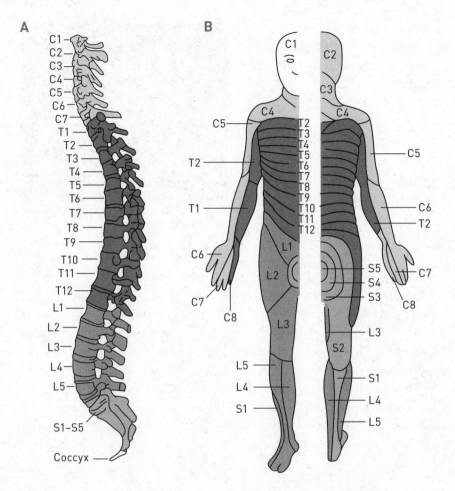

A

C1
C2
C3
C4
C5
C6
C7
T1
T2
T3
T4
T5
T6
T7
T8
T9
T10
T11
T12
L1
L2
L3
L4
L5
S1–S5
Coccyx

B

C1
C2
C3
C4
C5
T2
T3
T4
T5
T6
T7
T8
T9
T10
T11
T12
T2
T1
C6
L1
L2
C7
C8
L3
L5
L4
S1
C5
C6
T2
S5
S4
S3
C7
C8
L3
S2
S1
L4
L5

C

Level	Motor Function
C1–C4	Full paralysis of the limbs
C5	Paralysis of the wrists, hands, and triceps
C6	Paralysis of the wrist flexors, triceps, and hands
C7–C8	Some hand muscle weakness, difficulty grasping and releasing

Figure 2. The vertebrae, dermatomes, and associated functional deficits

and/or loss of sensation in all four limbs) or paraplegia (paralysis and/or loss of sensation only in the legs, usually). Paraplegia occurs when the injury is below T1. An SCI diagnosis is made by both clinical exam and imaging (Figure 3).

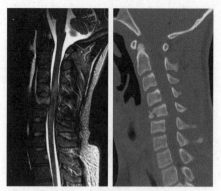

Figure 3: SCI with vertebrae damage and spinal cord contusion

Stroke: Stroke is a sudden loss of blood flow to a part of the brain, which causes cells to die. There are three major types of stroke (Figure 4): 1) ischemic, due to decreased blood flow from local blockage of a blood vessel; 2) embolic, due to decreased blood flow from a clot that travels up the carotid or vertebral artery; and 3) hemorrhagic, due to leakage or rupture of a blood vessel, causing bleeding into the brain. Stroke damage can resemble that of SCI because the death of cells in the part of the brain that senses or moves limbs can be similar. In the case of stroke, however, this usually occurs on only one side of your body. Stroke is also unique in that it can cause difficulty with speech (understanding or speaking language) or loss of vision on one side (rarely, TBI can have similar effects). A stroke diagnosis is made by both clinical exam and imaging.

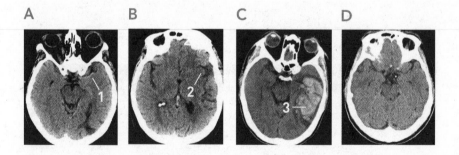

Figure 4: A. Embolic white line is an embolus stuck in a narrow vessel (1), B. Ischemic brain swelling due to lack of blood flow from embolus in (A) (2), C. Hemorrhagic Stroke blood in the brain from a leaking blood vessel (3), D. Normal

Traumatic Brain Injury (TBI): TBI (Figure 5) is damage to the brain resulting from an external mechanical force, such as the rapid acceleration and deceleration that occurs with a car accident or if your head hits a heavy object. Diagnosis can be easily made when the force causes bleeding or a skull fracture. Localized injuries are more frequent in TBI, and they are particularly common in the lower part of the frontal lobes, which are involved in "executive functions," such as social behavior, emotions, smell, and judgment. However, when the injury is widespread, there isn't much damage evident on a CT scan. Diffusion tensor imaging (DTI), which shows white matter tracts (the axons of the nerves) separate from the gray matter (the bodies of the nerves), is an excellent way to show diffuse damage. This appears as "white matter hyperintensities" (a starlike object in the deeper parts of the brain). Symptoms such as paralysis or difficulty with language may occur when the TBI is more severe.

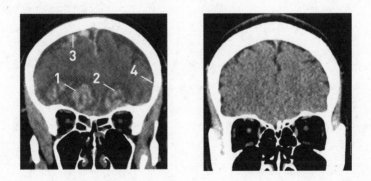

Figure 5: TBI showing frontal contusions (1 and 2), subdural hematoma (3), and traumatic subarachnoid hemorrhage (4) compared to normal (right)

The Autonomic Nervous System

The autonomic nervous system (ANS; Figure 6) is the main controller of your body's internal environment. It automatically maintains your blood pressure, heart rate, respiration, digestion, and body temperature. There are two major components: the sympathetic nervous system (SNS) and the parasympathetic nervous system (PNS). These work together and in opposition to control these functions every day. Unfortunately, damage to the brainstem or spinal cord disrupts the SNS and PNS, causing many problems. Chapters 9 through 14 discuss how damage to the ANS can make your life very difficult. Even worse, there are very few therapies to rehabilitate or restore it.

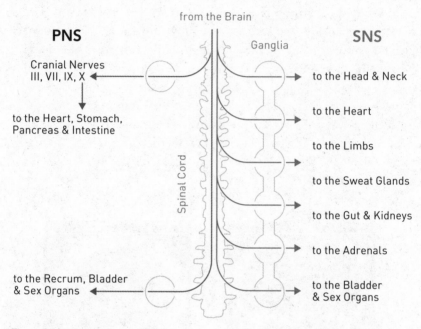

Figure 6. Autonomic nervous system

How This Book Can Help You

What you'll find in the pages ahead is everything I've learned—as a patient and as a doctor—about recovery after ANI. I'll take you from initial injury, through recovery, and all the way to leading your best life as an ANI survivor. You'll read about new devices, drugs, therapies, and approaches to "rewire" the brain that offer the possibility of actually *restoring* function. You'll also learn about the concept of neuroplasticity, the brain's ability to change how it performs a specific function by establishing new connections between nerves to restore these functions. Throughout it all, I'll remind you about the importance of goal setting, resilience, and tapping into the power of your mind.

One of the hardest parts of experiencing an ANI is the psychological trauma. Grappling with a "new normal" is profoundly difficult, mentally and emotionally. And, unlike a musculoskeletal injury, where the damage is visible, an ANI is hidden, and it often places an enormous burden on you and your family. Wrapping your mind around what you've experienced is the first step in your recovery, and this book contains advice to help you get there. This ability to deal with the psychological consequences of your injury not only starts your journey—it's also important every step of the way.

The information in this book is meant to educate and inspire you on your rehabilitation and recovery journey. It will show you the enormous variety of approaches to help you regain function. There are strong opinions on treatments to try and therapies to avoid. This isn't a prescription—it's a supplement to the recommendations of your medical team. Each person is unique, as is each ANI. Use what you learn in this book to have more in-depth conversations with your doctor and your therapy team.

Part 1 takes you through the initial injury and the power of your mind in the healing process. Part 2 shows you the vast landscape of neurorehabilitation and examines the similarities and differences between Western and Eastern medicine to provide multiple approaches to your recovery. Part 3 addresses many common medical problems you may face after ANI. In Part 4, you'll learn about adaptive devices that can help you enjoy a rewarding and meaningful life. And you'll learn about new and innovative therapies on the horizon and how to maintain your resilience despite years of disability. But first, we'll start at the beginning and learn how to deal with your initial grief, so you can start to heal.

Having an ANI is one of the most serious challenges anyone will face. Ultimately, what I've learned is that each day offers opportunities for joy. I hope this book will help you on your journey back to a meaningful life.

PART 1

Your Recovery Begins in Your Head

Battling the Blues

*How to Deal with Your Grief, Depression, and
Anxiety So You Can Focus on Recovery*

To SAY I HAD THE BLUES after the accident that paralyzed me would be an understatement. Before the accident, I had worked as CEO at a prestigious medical center; after the accident, I was unable to feed myself, go to the bathroom on my own, or even comb my hair. I had permanently lost the life I loved, and after the shock wore off, I was engulfed in grief.

Experiencing an ANI—whether it's a stroke, SCI, or TBI—is a profoundly life-changing event. The life you had is gone in an instant. And the awareness that your life will never be the same is inescapable. No matter how well your recovery goes, there will always be a distinction between *before* and *after*.

When you suffer an ANI, you've lost something that can't be retrieved. Your grief for that loss is as real as experiencing the death of a loved one, and it is to be *expected*, *acknowledged*, and *addressed with care*. And the sooner the better. It's the first important step in your rehabilitation.

But grief isn't the only mental health complication that may arise—and this is something that doctors often don't address. *At least* half of those who suffer an ANI experience depression, anxiety, and/or post-traumatic stress disorder (PTSD). I say at least half because the number is almost certainly higher. While these mental health disorders should be expected, too frequently the questions that would elicit your need for help are never asked. Why? Doctors and nurses often don't have this conversation because they believe it will take a long time. And it certainly does take a long time to arrive at an effective treatment; much of the therapy is hours-long one-on-one conversations and adjustments of medications, which may take months. And unfortunately, if left untreated, these conditions will greatly hamper your rehabilitation, degrading your quality of life as well as the lives of your loved ones.

There are two other related psychological health issues that can occur after ANI: 1) substance abuse, such as a dependence on narcotics and/or alcohol to numb painful thoughts, emotions, and memories, and 2) complicated grief, which is characterized by prolonged grieving and emotional instability (see page 26).

Further complicating the situation is that symptoms of these mental health disorders sometimes occur months *after* the accident, leaving you, your family, and your caregivers confused. But if you're prepared, you'll know how to ask for help. Addressing your mental health needs after ANI is *essential* to your functional recovery; without a sound mind, you can never restore a sound body.

Six Key Components of a Good Treatment Plan

There are six important points to keep in mind when it comes to finding a treatment plan that addresses your psychological needs:

- **Don't wait.** Think about the event that caused your grief, depression, anxiety, or PTSD as damage that requires immediate attention. Early intervention has major long-term benefits. Stated simply: The sooner you get mental health help, the sooner you can begin to rehabilitate effectively. If you stay in a state of shock or rapidly sink into depression, you lose a golden window of opportunity to regain function. If your medical team doesn't ask you about your emotional state, raise this topic with your doctor as soon as possible.

- **Call in the troops.** You'll need a multidisciplinary treatment plan to help address any mental health issues. Establish a coordinated network now; it will serve you well for many years. The team should include your primary care physician, your psychotherapist, a loved one who is responsible for your care and is in communication with your health care team, and a representative from the insurance company who addresses financial issues.

- **Mental health therapy works.** Psychotherapy—cognitive behavioral therapy (CBT) in particular—should be your default choice for treatment because it has no harmful side effects *and* it has been shown to be of significant benefit for people from all walks of life and for a variety of mental health disorders, including complicated grief, depression, anxiety, and PTSD.[1] To find a CBT therapist, ask your doctor and/or your close friends for recommendations.

- **Consider medications.** Medications will likely be necessary to deal with the mental health disorders that arise after an ANI. In fact, I recommend that people with an acute ANI be started on an antidepressant as soon as they are medically stable. More than 50 percent of ANI survivors will develop depression, and because it takes several weeks for most of these medications to become effective, valuable time for rehabilitation may be lost while the person experiences the consequences of depression, such as fatigue, lack of motivation, and difficulty sleeping. Combined with CBT, drugs can be incredibly effective at treating mental health disorders. It's also worth inquiring about other non-drug therapies that have shown to be highly effective, such as electroconvulsive therapy (ECT) and transcranial magnetic stimulation (TMS)[2]; see page 29 for more on these therapies.

- **Explore complementary medicine.** Complementary medicine treatments, which complement and strengthen the effects of modern Western medicine, include acupuncture, chiropractic treatment, hypnotherapy, massage, mindfulness, tai chi, and yoga. (You'll find out more about these therapies in chapter 8.)

- **Resilience and hope enable recovery.** Resilience means bending, not breaking, and then gradually coming back to a new equilibrium from adversity. It requires hope, the expectation that you *will* find new meaning for your life and recover enough function to enjoy it. Nurture your resilience and hope by enjoying as many of the activities that you enjoyed before your injury as possible. Perhaps that was spending time with family and friends, being outdoors, playing sports, reading, or praying. It's important to accept help that is offered (and make sure that you thank people for helping), while also reaching out for help when you need it. You may find hope and comfort by joining a support group or perhaps in the pages of this book.

Let's take a look now at how you can deal with your grief, depression, and anxiety so you can focus on recovery.

Grief

The best-known model of grief is the Kübler-Ross model, which moves from denial to anger, bargaining, depression, and, finally, to acceptance. Not everyone will experience all of these stages, and you may not experience them in this order. For ANI survivors, the process usually starts with *shock*, which is where we find ourselves before the grieving process can truly begin. It's important to recognize shock as an initial stage, so that you can allow yourself to grieve properly.

Shock

When I regained consciousness after my initial surgery, I found myself in a state of shock. I looked at my body and didn't recognize it. There was a tube in my nose, a breathing tube down my throat that prevented me from talking, a feeding tube that went into my stomach, a catheter in my bladder, and numerous intravenous lines. I wasn't able to move or feel below my neck, and I felt like I was floating in space with no sense of time or place. All of this made it difficult to know *who I was*, since I kept thinking about what I'd lost. I wondered about my future and was filled with fear and dread. I was mentally overwhelmed, and I couldn't even talk about it. Moving past the initial shock is different for everyone, but what helped me was communicating using a letter board (which allowed me to spell out words—a tedious and *slow* process), and my daughter Mariah's ability to read my lips. Later, small signs of progress, such as being able to move my left big toe, gave me something positive to focus on. As you work through recovery, hold on to these small signs—they could be what propels you out of your state of shock and allows you to begin the grieving process.

Denial

Most of us are not strangers to denial. With ANI, these feelings become a coping mechanism that serves to protect us from becoming overwhelmed by the enormity of our situation. But denial can be harmful if it persists because it prevents optimal rehabilitation and it can complicate therapy. If, for example, your feelings of denial about your condition cause you to think that you don't need psychological counseling, you are more likely to experience chronic grief and depression. To overcome denial, you must first acknowledge the reality of your situation. Your doctors, therapists, and friends can help—if you trust them, they will help you process the reality that you have experienced a major, life-changing event.

Anger

After ANI, feelings of anger can arise as an expression of intense frustration. It can be very frustrating for you to lose your independence and have to ask others for help. You may even be angry at yourself, blaming your actions for your injury. These are all very valid feelings, and you should allow yourself to take the time to feel them. But it's also important for you and your family to recognize that *sustained* anger will drive away the very people who can provide you with the greatest emotional assistance. A good therapist will help you address these feelings of anger from the start, before they become sustained and complicate your recovery. Because, when harnessed properly, anger can actually be a useful tool in the recovery process. I felt my loss of independence and self-reliance severely, but I was able to use that anger and frustration to work harder at my own rehabilitation.

Bargaining

If you are feeling particularly hopeless, you may find yourself turning to bargaining, thinking back to the events before your accident or even trying to make a deal with God. For me, this sounded like: *If only I had waited one minute longer before going down that hill, I wouldn't be in this situation.* This thought ran through my mind constantly. This is called *magical thinking*, and it serves to protect you from the weight of your grief after ANI. But it's not helpful to remain in this stage, nor is it based on an acceptance of your new reality. As you're going through it, know that you're not alone—it's a universal stage and can help you progress to the next one.

Depression

In the depression stage, you may feel sad, confused, and overwhelmed. Depression isn't limited to feelings of sadness, however; you may also feel physical symptoms, like fatigue or headache, and you may engage in destructive behaviors. It's not uncommon for people with depression to withdraw from social interactions for a period of time. For ANI survivors, this withdrawal can continue for years, becoming chronic depression. Being sad is a normal part of the process, but being depressed is a serious matter and not something to take lightly. But you don't have to live with your depression. If you find yourself in a sustained period of depression, seek support from your loved ones and treatment options from your primary care physician or therapist (refer to page 27 for more on this). You don't have to suffer alone.

Acceptance

Acceptance is the recognition that the loss of function due to your injury is likely to be permanent, but *some recovery is possible*. Acceptance is essential to beginning the process of functional recovery because it "ends" the grieving process and allows you to move into recovery. This doesn't mean there won't be setbacks, days when all you want to do is cry, but when combined with hope, acceptance enables you to maximize your physical and psychological recovery.

Whether your grief follows the Kübler-Ross model or a different path, you should take all the time you need to grieve, and you should be supported through your experience.

Complicated Grief

Diagnosis: If you're not able, for whatever reason, to experience your grief fully, you may develop complicated grief. Complicated grief becomes apparent when your feelings of loss do not lessen over time and become both mentally and physically debilitating, in some cases even leading to suicide.

Treatment: The best approach for treating complicated grief is cognitive behavioral therapy (CBT; see page 77). Together, the patient and therapist identify and discuss the recurring behaviors and thought patterns that have the person "stuck" in complicated grief. Then, the therapist works on strengthening key relationships that provide emotional support and on helping you visualize a future life. A CBT program will require three to four months of weekly therapy sessions and should be effective in about 70 percent of patients.[3] Therapy can help you move on, restoring a meaningful life in which you feel valuable to family, friends, and society.

I found that creating a mantra was very helpful in my healing. Mine is *forgive, let it go, move on*. At my toughest moments of recovery, repeating this mantra would help to calm me. I was able to make peace with my past by using the phrase *back in the day* as a shortcut for admitting to myself that I would never have the same abilities I had before my injury. Focusing on the positives helped—I could still perform a lot of the activities of daily life such as eating, brushing my teeth, and cooking (microwave only!). Of course, the mind can still play tricks: In my dreams, I'm never in a wheelchair!

Letting go of your past life is difficult, but it can be done. Once you're able to let go and accept your new life, you'll feel a weight lifted off your shoulders. Some families will want to honor that transition with a planned and meaningful acknowledgment that, ultimately, is all about showing the injured person that they are deeply loved. You may choose to celebrate your progress on the first anniversary of your injury.

Depression

Diagnosis: Depression is characterized by an increase in depressive feelings (sadness, emptiness, and hopelessness) and a decrease in pleasurable feelings (enjoyment of life, laughter, and happiness). Physicians make the clinical diagnosis of depression when these symptoms persist every day, for most of the day. Many patients suffer from undiagnosed depression, as doctors can't predict who will get depressed after an ANI. Surprisingly, for most ANI survivors, there is very little correlation between severity of your injury and depression. Depression can also be difficult to diagnose, since many who suffer from depression do so alone. There's a stigma associated with admitting depression, so many people are reluctant to talk about it.

Don't try to "tough it out" if you think you're depressed, or if a loved one thinks you are. When you do reach out to your doctor, don't be surprised if they evaluate you for other conditions that mimic depression or that can contribute to it, such as hypothyroidism, metabolic abnormalities (low calcium), anemia, and other infections (which can cause fatigue and lethargy). Your doctor may also address the possibility that side effects of your medications may be causing your depression.

Treatment: The American Psychiatric Association recommends that initial treatment be individualized, so you should work together with your loved ones and your medical team to determine the best treatment for you. Factors that can influence the choice of treatment include the severity of symptoms, coexisting disorders, prior treatment experience, cost, duration of treatment, and patient preference. Options include cognitive behavioral therapy (CBT), drug treatment, electroconvulsive therapy (ECT; see page 29), transcranial magnetic stimulation (TMS; see page 30), exercise, and complementary medicine (see page 118).

CBT is often the best treatment for depression. If you are depressed—feeling worthless and helpless every time you spill something while trying to eat, for example—CBT helps you to be open to the process of learning rather than getting frustrated. Through role-playing conversations with your therapist, you can learn how to have an argument, for example, without being swamped by feelings of self-pity or worthlessness. Techniques that support what you learn in CBT—meditation, mindfulness, and relaxation behaviors, such as slowing your breathing—can also be helpful in treatment for depression.

Antidepressant medication is frequently recommended as an initial treatment choice for depression, often in tandem with CBT or other types of psychotherapy. There are three classes of drugs for this treatment: selective serotonin reuptake inhibitors (SSRIs), serotonin-norepinephrine reuptake inhibitors (SNRIs), and tricyclic antidepressants (TCAs). It's important that your medical doctor and your therapist have a strong working relationship, as many of the drugs have significant side effects. If you develop adverse side effects, make sure that you contact the doctor who prescribed the medication and that the nature of the side effect is listed in your medical record.

Drug therapy for depression is slow in onset, requiring up to four weeks to show signs of improvement, with maximal benefit requiring as many as twelve weeks. Your doctor may choose to start you on an SSRI, which will increase serotonin levels in the brain, or an SNRI, which will increase both serotonin and norepinephrine levels. Both types of drugs can have significant side effects, so it's important to be aware of these before you start taking them. SSRIs are associated with nausea, anorexia, diarrhea, insomnia, agitation, and anxiety, and each SSRI has unique side effects with respect to issues such as sedation, constipation, sexual dysfunction, and weight gain. SNRIs have a broader range of potential treatments and may be slightly more effective. This is particularly true for people who also have anxiety, since the brain receptors inhibited by the SNRIs are thought to include some that mediate fear and worry. If the

Early Treatment of Depression

Starting antidepressants soon after injury may prevent later depression. This theory has been most extensively studied for stroke, and the American Heart Association recommends beginning therapy with an SSRI when you are medically stable, about one week after your event.[4] There are no reliable clinical data on early use of SSRIs for TBI and SCI survivors, but because depression is common in these conditions as well, there may be benefit in early treatment.

There have been several clinical trials to treat depression using anti-inflammatory drugs, particularly for Celebrex (celecoxib), which is a nonsteroidal anti-inflammatory drug (NSAID). Results from these trials appear to show a significant benefit in treating depression.[5] NSAIDs such as Celebrex, however, have been associated with hypertension and increased risk of heart attack—risks that need to be weighed against potential benefit. This is particularly true for stroke patients, since many of the risk factors for stroke are similar to those associated with heart attack.

drug is effective, your doctor should continue treatment for at least six months after your symptoms have improved. If the drug is not effective, you can switch more easily to an alternative within the same type, before switching to one from another type. If SSRIs and SNRIs don't offer relief, your doctor may prescribe a TCA. Though TCAs are significantly less expensive, they are substantially more likely to cause symptoms such as dry mouth, constipation, dizziness, sweating, and blurred vision, and the consequences of overdose are much more serious.

Brain Activation Procedures: For patients who do not improve significantly with psychotherapy, CBT, and/or medications, there are a number of noninvasive procedures that use electrical and magnetic fields to modify brain function. These are referred to as neuromodulation, and the two most common types are electroconvulsive therapy (ECT) and repetitive transcranial magnetic stimulation (rTMS).

ECT is the most effective neuromodulation therapy for depression. It uses an electrical current discharged between two electrodes on the scalp to induce a generalized seizure. The typical therapy is three shocks each week for two to four weeks. Usually, an antidepressant is used in combination with ECT, since the benefit is greater than using either one alone. It's also associated with potentially serious side effects and safety risks, such as transient amnesia and occasional memory loss, headache, and cardiovascular problems—the latter, such as low heart rate, are common but very short lasting. However, in people with cardiac disease (frequent in people with stroke), there is a 10 percent complication rate, including chest pain, abnormal heart rhythm, and decreased blood flow to parts of the heart (ischemia). Because of these problems, ECT is less popular than other types of therapy.

rTMS uses electricity passing through a metal coil to generate a magnetic field that activates nerve cells in the brain. A typical course of rTMS therapy is a daily treatment for four weeks. Though it's not as effective as ECT and has a relatively high relapse rate, most patients prefer rTMS because there's no seizure involved, and it's safer than ECT.[6]

Exercise: Exercise has been shown to provide significant benefits as a treatment for depression.[7] Work with your physical therapy team to design an exercise plan that is suited to your abilities. Important rules for exercise include: 1) Go slowly so you don't hurt yourself. I didn't realize how easy it was to get injured while exercising after my injury. Because my sensation is poor, I could twist an ankle or strain a muscle and not know it until the next day when a bruise appeared. 2) Work with your occupational therapists and physical therapists to develop stretching and strengthening programs that complement your functional needs. For the first three months after I returned home, my exercise consisted of getting out of bed and dressing, going to work, physical therapy for thirty minutes every day, and finally getting into bed at night. All of this was done with assistance, and it still left me exhausted!

> ### Exercise
> Exercise after stroke and TBI must be prescribed carefully because it may decrease blood flow to the damaged brain and worsen long-term recovery. Your doctor will advise you and your physical therapist how much exercise you should perform and what symptoms indicate potential harm.

Anxiety Disorders

Anxiety disorders, such as general anxiety, panic attacks, and PTSD, are characterized by feelings of anxiety and fear, where anxiety is a recurring worry about future events, and fear is a reaction to current events.[8] After your injury, you may have many new fears—it's very common, for example, to develop a fear of falling. Other issues that can cause anxiety include loss of independence, financial hardships, difficulties in interpersonal relationships, and concerns about bowel and bladder accidents.

Diagnosis: Anxiety is usually apparent during a clinical examination, although many patients are reluctant to talk about their fears. That's why it's important for your health care providers to speak to both you and your loved ones about your mental health. You may have anxiety if you find yourself avoiding an activity, feeling sick or tired prior to an activity, or crying in anticipation of an activity. Other symptoms are highly individual; for example, my anxiety is usually associated with becoming irritable, and even angry.

Treatment: Similar to treating depression, treatment of anxiety typically involves both therapy and medications. CBT is the approach most commonly used for anxiety because it helps you understand what makes you anxious and fearful, and provides training in how to adjust your response so that your symptoms become less severe.[9] One effective treatment for anxiety is "repeated exposure," in which you are repeatedly exposed to images that make you anxious. With the help of a therapist you will learn relaxation techniques to help you manage your anxiety. Over time you will develop "immunity" to the images as the exposure time is increased. As with depression, SSRIs and SNRIs are the first-choice medications for anxiety.

Acute Stress Disorder (ASD) and Post-Traumatic Stress Disorder (PTSD)

Diagnosis: ASD and PTSD are diagnosed by symptoms that involve reliving or avoiding the traumatic event associated with the injury. The difference between ASD and PTSD is simply time: ASD occurs within one month of the traumatic event, and the symptoms of PTSD extend beyond that first month. Patients with ASD or PTSD can exhibit two very different behavioral responses: They can become agitated when exposed to someone or something in the environment that causes them to reexperience the trauma, or they can withdraw from the environment and become numb to the situation. Symptoms include flashbacks, nightmares, trouble concentrating, irritability, and depression.

My PTSD

I realized I was suffering from symptoms of PTSD about eighteen months after my initial injury. Several times in the first six months after my injury, I would reexperience the shock of my accident whenever I felt unexpected pain. Once, when a nurse was using a lift device to transfer me from my chair to bed, I felt pain that shot up my arm into my shoulder. Without conscious thought, I screamed as loud as possible, started swearing, and then began to sob uncontrollably. Similar reactions occurred every month or so during the first two years after my injury, but because these reactions occurred so infrequently, I didn't talk to my doctor.

I also suffered two recurring nightmares. The first was hitting my head against a low-hanging beam while in a friend's house. The other was being trapped in a house in which there were no clean or well-functioning toilets. These nightmares would usually wake me up at 4:30 in the morning, after which I could not go back to sleep. My PTSD has improved over time, through a combination of improved pain control and CBT.

Treatment: It's important to treat PTSD aggressively, since it has been associated with cancer, arthritis, digestive disease, and cardiovascular disease (it can increase the risk of hypertension, heart attack, and stroke).[10] PTSD is normally treated with CBT alone, especially with exposure therapy to decrease agitation and improve mood. Exposure therapy with CBT is usually quite intense and requires a period of three to four months. Drug therapies are quite effective in decreasing the symptoms of agitation and mood (irritability, anger, depression). Since PTSD is a type of anxiety, SSRIs are the first-line drugs, followed by SNRIs. There are a number of small but meaningful studies of complementary medicine therapies, such as acupuncture, yoga, and meditation, that show benefits in preventing and treating anxiety and stress disorders (you'll find more on this in chapter 8). Let your health care team know that you'd like to investigate the options that appeal to you.

Treating PTSD-associated sleep problems is crucial, since poor sleep can contribute further to PTSD symptoms and can slow healing and recovery. There's good evidence that CBT can address sleep disturbances. As always, treatment is highly individualized, and any decisions about how to address your sleep problems should be based on a conversation with your doctor.

Substance Abuse

In speaking with ANI survivors over the last ten years, I have found that many of them abuse alcohol or are addicted to pain medications, especially opiates (e.g., fentanyl, codeine, oxycodone, and hydrocodone). Social drinking is part of American culture. Yet most adults can't define a "standard drink." Why does that matter? Because you may already be in the habit of drinking enough on a daily or weekly basis for you to qualify as a person with a drinking problem. A standard drink is one glass (5 ounces/150 ml) of wine, one can or bottle (12 ounces/350 ml) of beer, or one shot (1.5 ounces/45 ml) of 80 proof hard liquor. Moderate alcohol consumption for healthy adults typically means up to one drink per day for women and two drinks per day for men.

Diagnosis: A two-question screening test for excess alcohol consumption is: "Do you sometimes drink beer, wine, or other alcoholic beverages?" and "How many times in the past year have you had four (for women) to five (for men) or more drinks in a day?"[11] If the answer is "Yes" to consumption, and "Yes" to four or five drinks, there is an 80 percent chance that you have "unhealthy alcohol use."

It can be difficult to differentiate between abuse and therapeutic use of drugs because many of the addictive drugs also successfully address ANI-related pain. Substance abuse and addiction are major health problems for anyone, but particularly for ANI survivors, because these drugs can have toxic effects on your physical health (they can contribute to cardiovascular disease and pressure ulcers), and your mental health (they can cause depression and suicide). If you or your family are concerned that your use of alcohol and opiates may qualify as abuse, you should have a discussion with your doctor. Don't put this conversation off for fear of being judged; substance abuse problems are quite common, and getting help can transform your quality of life.

Alcohol and TBI

Fifty percent of TBIs are associated with alcohol abuse—either in the person causing the injury or in the injured person. TBI survivors are also especially sensitive to alcohol, so most physicians recommend no alcohol for one year after injury.

Treatment: There are three major treatment approaches for substance abuse: 1) a continuing-care model for chronic disease, 2) medications, and 3) therapy. As part of your treatment, your doctor may also recommend support groups like Alcoholics Anonymous (AA) and Narcotics Anonymous (NA).

1. **Continuing-care model:** Any type of substance abuse treatment should include routine assessment and ongoing monitoring, because individuals with substance abuse frequently have a lifelong problem of periods of abstinence followed by periods of abuse. It's estimated that up to 60 percent of patients treated for alcohol or other drug abuse relapse within a year after treatment. Therefore, the treatment plan should be individualized and based on the severity of the abuse, the person's overall health, and the level of external support. Key elements of a treatment plan include having the patient take responsibility for managing the problem, providing links to other sources of support, and ongoing monitoring of drug and/or alcohol use.

2. **Medications:** For opiate addiction, drugs such as methadone and buprenorphine are effective for withdrawal symptoms and staying drug-free. Both drugs work by eliminating withdrawal symptoms and relieving drug cravings without producing a "high." For alcoholics who fail to stay sober with CBT or other psychotherapy, medications such as naltrexone and acamprosate can be beneficial.

3. **Therapy and support groups:** One of the most effective treatment approaches is combining traditional therapies, such as CBT, with support groups, like Alcoholics Anonymous (AA). These programs include mentorship (frequently by a former substance abuser), enjoyable alcohol- and drug-free social activities, and frequent support meetings. For many, these are the most effective (and certainly the least expensive) treatments, because of the social support network they create.

Social Support

Since it can be difficult for ANI survivors to attend AA or NA meetings, you may find support and community at injury-specific meetings. I know that this is particularly true in the SCI group, where wheelchair social events are well-attended, not only to exchange information (especially for "newbies"), but also to help find physicians and other health professionals for treatment of ongoing medical and psychiatric problems. We share a strong bond that facilitates long-term maintenance of abstinence.

Psychosocial Network (Your Support System)

A strong psychosocial network is a critical ingredient in mental health care, particularly during recovery from an injury or traumatic event. The links in the chain of your support network are all vulnerable after ANI, so paying attention to the potential pitfalls is important.

- **Spouse:** Spouses are usually the family member most impacted by ANI, because they may have to assume new responsibilities, many of which they're not prepared for. It's critical for the healthy spouse to make the time to focus on being a *companion and partner*, while remaining an independent person with their own interests. If your finances limit your ability to hire outside help, ask other family members to assist. But be very careful as you navigate this new normal. Spouses who become full-time caregivers are likely to experience anger, anxiety, and difficulties with intimacy, often leading to divorce. Underlying problems in the marriage become more pronounced. In particular, disagreements over money may become more intense, because of the increased expenses for medical care. While it may be difficult to discuss, intimacy is essential in maintaining the integrity of the marriage (more on this in chapter 7).

- **Family and friends:** In the first few weeks after your injury, family and friends may be galvanized to help and will likely appear in large numbers at the hospital. Interest usually wanes over time, though, especially if your hospital stay lasts several months. By the time you are discharged, only your spouse, children, and parents are likely to visit routinely. It can be hard to feel like your loved ones don't support you, but try not to be judgmental of friends and family who don't come to the hospital; many of them may simply feel uncomfortable seeing you so gravely ill. Even once you return home, visits from loved ones may occur infrequently, perhaps limited to weekends or holidays. Remember that your loved ones have their own families, spouses, and careers, and try not to take it personally.

  It's important that everyone who is actively involved in the care and recovery therapies continue to maintain their *own* physical, social, and emotional health. In the first year after injury, family counseling is an excellent way to work through this new, emotionally charged life situation. There are support groups for loved ones of ANI survivors that promote socialization, exchange of information about treatment options, and identification of health care providers with expertise in specific areas. These groups can be especially valuable for family members, allowing them to see the diversity of recovery in different individuals and to make new friends who understand their experience. Ask your doctor for a list of support groups in your area.

- **Finances:** It is the unfortunate reality of American health care that long-term medical care is expensive and frequently not covered fully by insurance policies. And if you have limited financial resources, the only way to receive this necessary health care is to apply for Social Security Disability Insurance for Medicaid or Medicare coverage. This can mean you will have access to a limited choice of doctors (some physicians will not accept Medicaid or Medicare patients, because reimbursement is significantly lower than for patients with commercial insurance).

  Early on, it's important to develop a long-term budget for care. I hired a life planner to create a plan for me based on my life expectancy. She was a former registered nurse who had worked with ANI patients both in hospitals and in ambulatory settings. While hiring a life planner is expensive ($1,000 to $2,000, depending on your specific circumstances), the calculations she provided gave me a sense of security by showing me what financial resources I would need over my expected lifespan. If your finances do not allow for the services of a life planner, have someone on your team investigate free financial counseling, which may be available at your local community center or offered pro bono by local advisory groups.

- **Health care system:** In many health care systems (networks that include hospitals, outpatient rehab centers, labs, diagnostic imaging, ambulatory surgical centers, visiting nurse agencies, and physician groups), there is a comprehensive plan for discharge, rehabilitation, and long-term care to ensure maximal independence, prevent readmission to the hospital, and promote efficient use of medical resources for the patient and the hospital.

  In the *advanced medical home model* (also known as the *patient-centered medical home model*), the primary care physician, working with other health providers, coordinates all aspects of patient care. This means that the providers (including social workers, rehabilitation counselors, and case managers) manage both the patient's medical *and* psychosocial issues. After ANI, I believe that team should also include palliative care specialists, who focus on quality of life. Palliative care providers integrate the psychological and spiritual aspects of a patient's care, with a focus on mental wellness. Palliative care social workers are trained to help address financial matters as well.

Now that you have the skills to handle grief, anxiety, and depression, you can learn to use your mind productively to rehabilitate and restore your body and regain the functions that you've lost. In the next chapter, you'll learn how to prepare for your discharge so that you can live as independently as possible as you continue your rehabilitation.

———

Everything You Need to Know

ANI is a major trauma that affects every aspect of your life. Let yourself grieve. It's important that you acknowledge and address your grief, and that of your loved ones, so that you can move forward in recovery. Unresolved grief (or complicated grief) can create disabling mental health disorders.

- Mental health disorders such as depression, anxiety, and PTSD are common after ANI. They should be expected and approached proactively.

- Remaining hopeful and resilient can have immeasurably positive influences on your recovery. Be sure to tap into the things that nurture your strength, and don't be afraid to lean on your support network. They want you to!

- There are a multitude of effective treatment approaches for grief, depression, anxiety, and PTSD. The most common are cognitive behavioral therapy (CBT) and medications: SSRIs, like citalopram (Celexa), escitalopram (Lexapro), fluoxetine (Prozac), paroxetine

(Paxil), and sertraline (Zoloft); and SNRIs, like duloxetine (Cymbalta), tramadol (Ultram), and venlafaxine (Effexor XR). These can be used in conjunction with older drugs like nortriptyline, to decrease dose and lessen side effects while improving pain control. Early intervention with both CBT and drugs may have the most benefit.

- A multidisciplinary team approach, anchored by your primary care physician, is essential to address the psychological and medical problems associated with ANI. Be sure to ask for palliative care if it is not offered.

- Planning for and taking advantage of resources outside of the hospital are critical for successful transition to a new life. Your social network of providers, family, and friends needs to be as strong as possible. Find support groups and get a referral to a family counselor. Group family therapy during the first year after ANI can be extremely helpful.

- Discuss carefully with your physician the use of any new mental health therapies, and weigh the risks and the benefits. You should only continue to use therapies if they are beneficial to you.

The Amazing Connection Between Your Mind and Body

How to Harness the Power of Your Mind with
Neuroplasticity for Optimal Recovery

AFTER MY ACCIDENT, I spent ten days in the intensive care unit at Strong Memorial Hospital in Rochester before I was transferred to the Kessler Rehabilitation Center in New Jersey, a hospital that specializes in spinal cord injury rehabilitation. I was still on a ventilator, which meant I was unable to speak. I was paralyzed and terrified at the thought of leaving the town, colleagues, and medical center I knew so well. I was lucky that my wife was able to come with me and stay in a nearby apartment that belonged to friends of ours who were away for the summer. I was also fortunate that my twenty-six-year-old son lived in Jersey City, New Jersey, about thirty minutes away from the hospital. He had a full-time job, but he visited every Wednesday night for dinner and on most weekends.

Physical therapy at Kessler began the day after I arrived—yes, even while I was on the ventilator. Gradually, I was weaned off the ventilator and my physical therapy continued, increasing in duration and difficulty. One hundred days would pass before I left the rehab center and returned home to Rochester. Every morning at Kessler when I awoke, I was reminded anew of the reality of my injuries, how dramatically my life had changed, and how uncertain my future was. The weight of that awareness was suffocating. It took every ounce of mental fortitude I could muster to face each day. During my recovery, I found three mental tools essential in helping me regain function.

The Three Essential Mental Tools for Recovery

The expression "sound mind, sound body" is never more relevant than for individuals recovering from an ANI. To get your brain and body back takes more than courage. Although you and your loved ones will need plenty of that, you will also need to use the *mental* tools that make recovery possible. The three essential mental qualities you need to tap into are:

Resilience: Your belief in yourself and your ability to get through tough times. Resilience can be bolstered by your spiritual faith or by recalling how you overcame earlier challenges in life.

Focus: Focus is essential to anything important that you want to accomplish in life, and that's especially true when it comes to the hard work it will take for you to achieve your goals after your injury.

Persistence: To take advantage of neuroplasticity and rewire your brain in ways that allow your body to perform functions that were lost by your injury, you must practice hundreds of times to become an expert. Because the path to expertise is not a straight line, you must be determined to achieve your goals, large and small, on your way to recovery; and persist during periods of little to no progress.

You and your loved ones can develop these mental qualities as individuals and as a team. They overlap and connect, each one strengthening the others. Let's take a closer look.

Resilience

There are four essential components of resilience.

1. A belief that we control our response to adversity

2. Confidence that we can develop new approaches to solving our problems

3. Perseverance: Resilience is more than a glass-half-full attitude. In fact, one must face the negatives of a situation to be able to address them and develop solutions.

4. A team effort: Trying to do everything on your own, without asking for help, makes recovering from your injury much more difficult. Don't go it alone.

The founding director of the Resilience Project, Hugh van Cuylenburg, cites three attitudes—gratitude, empathy, and mindfulness—that develop and strengthen resilience.[1] Here are the behaviors that helped me on my journey to becoming more resilient.

Gratitude: To cultivate gratitude, keep a gratitude journal. Every evening, write down three positive things that happened during the day. Write about the best thing that happened to you, the person for whom you are most grateful and why, and what you're looking forward to most about tomorrow. Studies show that within six weeks of keeping a daily gratitude journal, patients experience physical *and* mental improvements in their lives—better sleep, improved immunity, increased feelings of happiness, and fewer symptoms of depression and anxiety.[2]

Empathy: Every time you do something kind for someone else, your brain releases molecules called neurotransmitters that make you feel happier, more energetic, and more positive. In recovery, I realized empathy was a crucial skill that I needed to practice. No matter how severe my injury was, there was always someone "worse off" than me. I would routinely spend time with others to learn about their struggles and let them know that I understood how difficult it was to be in their situation. It's important to be able to listen and understand without the need to provide advice.

I also discovered that my caregivers responded very positively to empathy. Early after my injury, I was very inwardly focused and didn't think of my caregivers as having lives outside of the hospital. But I can't stress enough how important it is, for both you and them, to be empathetic to your caregivers. They'll respond positively to your taking an interest in them as people. Plus, being empathetic will make you feel better and more confident in your ability to help others.

Mindfulness: The ability to be completely present in the moment in a nonjudgmental state is the essence of mindfulness. Learning how to be mindful—through classes, books, apps, and more—helps you maintain focus on one task and be fully in the moment, whether it's having a conversation, writing a letter, or participating in a sport. Mindfulness also teaches you to be more self-aware. This is a powerful tool to facilitate your mental and physical recovery because it keeps you from *catastrophic thinking*—unrelenting negative mental fretting about what-if scenarios.

Focus

Focus is the ability to be simultaneously aware of your environment and concentrate on a specific task, using all your abilities to accomplish it. You've likely heard the phrase "wrapping your mind around the problem," but how do you do that intentionally, regularly, and with positive results? Believe it or not, there's a method that teaches you how to do this and therapies that can help you focus on achieving results. Athletes frequently refer to this method as "getting in the zone." It's a state of mind where you are relaxed but completely focused on the demands you ask of your body. Much of this involves practice and repetition, combined with an intense concentration on the present situation.

A good example of focus was my approach to improving my walking. The key ingredients were coaching by my physical therapist, watching YouTube videos on proper walking technique by both disabled and nondisabled people, and total concentration. The first step in focusing is to learn what skills you must master to achieve your goal. For me to improve my walking, this included a wider stance, a consistent heel strike followed by pushing off with my toes, an upright posture, and use of the gluteus maximus muscles (the big ones in your butt) to push forward. Learning each skill took several weeks, and integrating them together took several years! But the results have been gratifying compared to when I started—today, I can walk ten times farther and at least twice as fast.

To strengthen your ability to focus, you need an organized approach. You have to make a dedicated time commitment (it's best to make it the same time every day), be in the right environment, and have a good teacher. Every day when I go to work, I schedule my three rehabilitation activities—walking, standing, and exercising on my bicycle—to ensure that I have time to complete them. In terms of environment, convenience is important. For example, I stand and cycle in my office using a computer and external monitor to enable me to work while I exercise. And, when I walk, there are no distractions. My physical therapist, assistant, and I are quiet, except when they comment on my technique.

Persistence

To achieve your goals, you need the determination to persevere. For example, learning how to walk again requires that you break the goal into component skills that you will practice hundreds of times. This can be both boring and frustrating, especially since progress is rarely linear, with successes followed by long plateaus. It is during these times of no progress that you may want to stop trying, but persistence will carry you through. At times, you may not be able to practice because of injuries and other health issues. It's crucial that you keep going at some level, especially during times of extreme hardship. A good friend told me that the hardest time of his rehabilitation was when he developed a pressure ulcer (more on this in chapter 13) and had to lie in bed for twenty hours each day until it healed. As a result, he lost much of the progress he had made in recovery and needed to start all over again, but persistence carried him through.

How to Harness the Power of Your Mind

There are three concepts critical to this idea:

1. If the mind is a mental concept, and not physical, how does it interact with the brain? The brain is a physical object composed of 14 to 16 billion nerves and even more additional cell types, while the mind represents the product of the brain's nerve activity, thinking. Thinking has been translated into something measurable by doctors, the state of consciousness, which is measured by the Glasgow Coma Scale (GCS, see Table 1). The GCS measures consciousness by the level of stimulation required to cause the person to open their eyes, respond to speech, and move in response to pain. Each response is graded from 1 to 5, so the lowest total score is 3 (indicating deep unconsciousness) and the highest is 15 (indicating fully awake). Importantly, the admission GCS has been

Eye Opening	Score
Spontaneous	4
Response to verbal command	3
Response to pain	2
No eye opening	1
Best Verbal Response	**Score**
Oriented	5
Confused	4
Inappropriate words	3
Incomprehensible sounds	2
No verbal response	1
Best Motor Response	**Score**
Obeys commands	6
Localizing response to pain	5
Withdrawal response to pain	4
Flexion to pain	3
Extension to pain	2
No motor response	1
Total normal (fully conscious)	15

Table 1: Glasgow Coma Scale

linked to prognosis for ANI, especially TBI (scores of 3 to 5 are associated with very poor outcomes).

2. Neuroplasticity is the ability of the brain to "rewire" itself by building new connections between nerves. When the brain is damaged, the mind has to find another way to perform a task. This process occurs through visualization. Your mind visualizes how your body will perform a task, and your brain executes the appropriate commands.

3. Practice is critical to neurorestoration. I practiced lifting plastic wine glasses thousands of times and then practiced another thousand times with increasing amounts of water in the glass, all before I was able to try lifting real wine in a real glass.

Neuroplasticity

Neuroplasticity is most apparent in stroke survivors. If a stroke occurs in the right side of the brain, 1,500 of the 30,000 genes that make up the DNA of the cells in the damaged right side of the brain are altered, but more genes change (2,000 out of 30,000) on the uninjured left side of the brain. This is clearly a compensation by the left side of the brain to help the damaged right side.

My story is simple. I was right-handed before my SCI, but after the injury, my left arm and hand were four times stronger and had a range of motion three times greater than that of my right arm and hand. So I trained myself to be left-handed by visualizing how it should move. Now I can pour a glass of wine and drink it left-handed, which I could not do previously.

Neuroplasticity

Neuroplasticity has three parts: learning, compensation, and recovery.[3]

1. Learning is the process of acquiring knowledge, behaviors, and skills through experience or study, or by being taught.

2. Compensation occurs when a part of the brain that isn't injured takes over the function of the injured part.

3. Recovery is improvement of function in an injured area. The body's synapses (connections between nerve cells) can increase to change the quality and quantity of their interactions. This reorganization is likely dependent on learning and compensation, along with a heavy dose of practice.

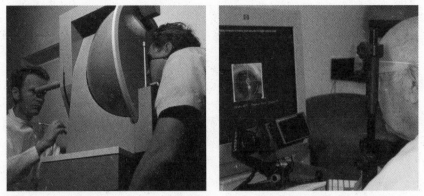

Figure 7: Visual training to restore some of the basic vision lost to TBI and stroke

For example, if you've lost your ability to see the left side of your visual field after a stroke, you can regain some of this vision by practicing a phenomenon called *blindsight*, since you likely have visual neurons that are still alive.[4] These neurons can be activated in a coordinated fashion by repetitive practice—in this case, by staring intently into a white globe with a red laser dot shining into it (Figure 7). The technician flashes the laser in several places and asks you to signal when you see it. Initially, you may see it only in one or two places, but over many hours of practice, you will steadily see it more often in the part of your visual field next to your blind spot. Through repeated practice of this activity, the living visual neurons form new synapses. Further neuroplasticity occurs by uninjured parts of the brain that exist outside of the visual cortex joining via unknown mechanisms. In most patients this "reassembled" visual sensor generates a stimulus (sufficient electrical activity) of the visual field to be detected by your brain.

The key principle in this process is that recovery and compensation depend on nerve cells being recruited to form new synapses. This is called the Hebbian theory,[5] which describes how brain neurons change during the learning process. Simply put, "neurons that fire together, wire together," or new connections between nerves that are used frequently become more stable and recruit additional nerves to form a new mature pathway. In this way, repetitive firing of newly formed synapses creates new groups of neurons that compensate for lost function. For example, I now use my left hand to pour a glass of wine and drink from it, when I was right-handed all my life. For people with ANI, this offers a clear path to recovery. In chapter 19 we'll look at several ways that new technologies take advantage of this principle to promote functional recovery.

Rehabilitation and Neuroplasticity

Rehabilitation is focused on restoring physical functions. It teaches your brain how to compensate by altering your behavior, or how to restore function by improving the lost function itself. For example, teaching someone how to use a cane or a buttonhook is a compensatory behavioral approach for a neurological problem such as a weak leg or a lack of dexterity and strength in your fingers. It may also include work-around solutions or substitute skills, such as teaching people with right arm and hand paralysis to tie shoes using only the left arm and hand.

Restoration of function is much more difficult than recovery of function. Restoration of function involves restoring neurons at the site of damage to normal function or causing new cells to grow and differentiate into neurons (the hope of stem cell therapy). Recovery of function means that you can perform the task, but it frequently requires use of other nerves located outside the previous pathway. Both processes require repetitive use and stimulation of the paralyzed limb. To master a task that requires "*restorative* neuroplasticity," Peter G. Levine, author of *Stronger After Stroke*, identified four components.[6]

1. **Repetition.** Mastering a movement requires hundreds, if not thousands, of repetitions; such as described above for visual restoration using blindsight.

2. **Task-specific.** It's easier to rewire the brain if the task is "real world." If you're a painter attempting the "reach and grasp" task, for example; it's much better if your goal is to grasp a paint brush, rather than a child's block (an object typically used in adult occupational therapy).

3. **Massed practice.** The repetition and task-specific practice should occur in time-intensive sessions; two to three hours a day for one to two weeks, for example, rather than one to two hours every other day for one to two months. This time dedication may not be possible for people who work full-time jobs, as I currently do. But I was able to follow the massed practice model when I took a leave of absence to travel to China several years ago. For eight weeks, I performed neurorehabilitation six days a week for seven hours a day. There, I made the greatest progress ever in my overall health, strength, body control, and task-specific skills. (More about this in chapter 8.)

4. **Novel or challenging tasks.** Practice tasks that are new or difficult for you. For example, I progressed from being hand-fed by an aide (since I could only lift my arm to my mouth twice before I became exhausted), to drinking from a sippy-cup or lifting food with a modified spoon or fork, and finally to drinking from a stemmed wine glass and cutting meat with a knife and fork.

Common Neuroplasticity Exercises

Mirror box exercise

One of the oldest therapies for neurorehabilitation of the upper extremity is the mirror box (Figure 8). You place the paralyzed or weak arm and hand inside the box and the functioning arm and hand outside the box, so that you can see it reflected in the mirror. When you rotate the functioning hand, it looks like the paralyzed hand. If

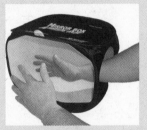

you rotate both hands at the same time it looks, to your brain, like the paralyzed limb is moving. Repetition is key here: When done hundreds of times, this exercise can strengthen the paralyzed limb. As the limb becomes stronger, the process can be targeted to a specific task. If the task has personal meaning, the extra motivation can strengthen your perseverance to repeat the exercise.

Figure 8: Mirror box

The BIONIK InMotionARM

To develop accuracy and strength for my reach and grasp, I used a state-of-the-art robot that was designed for the arm and hand (Figure 9). This robot has sophisticated analysis tools, which allow you and your therapist to see exactly how many repetitions you did, at what speed, and with what level of strength and accuracy.

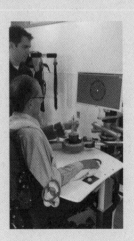

Figure 9: BIONIK InMotionARM

There were two tasks I practiced extensively. The first was the wagon wheel. In this exercise, you move the joystick from the center to the lighted circle at the rim while trying to stay on the spoke and move as fast as possible. The baseline test is to perform one circle of eight "out and back" movements against no resistance (Figure 10). This is much harder than it sounds, because it's easy for the hand to wander. It reminds me of figure skaters tracing circular patterns on the ice.

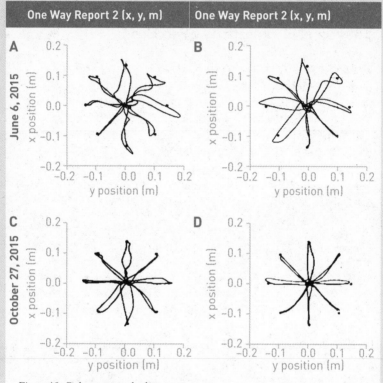

Figure 10. Robot wagon wheel progress

After the baseline test, I would perform the exercise by repeating the out-and-back movement eighty times, then resting for one to two minutes and repeating the exercise three more times, for a total of 320 movements. As shown (compare 10B & D to 10A & C), there was an obvious improvement in my speed and accuracy after the exercise. Because of my schedule, I could spend only one hour, three times a week, using the robot. But I still made rapid progress in just four months (compare 10D to 10B)—I was able to move in straighter lines, which I performed 50 percent faster. While not as effective as massed practice, this was sufficient repetition to show measured improvement. This translated into better dexterity for eating, typing, and handling objects, such as my phone.

I also performed a strengthening exercise in which the robot tried to pull me off the center hub every two seconds for two minutes. Over the first six months, I made significant progress in strength; the robot's ability to move me off the center hub was reduced by 50 percent. My strength improved to a level that enabled me to hold my coffee mug with my right hand and twist the top with my left hand to open it.

It should be noted that not all neuroplasticity is beneficial. Many ANI survivors have chronic pain in their paralyzed limb because the mind interprets the loss of information (both sensation and movement) as pain. I experienced an increase in pain in the biceps of my right arm two years after my original injury. This progressed to complex regional pain syndrome (CRPS; see page 83), in which I had changes in blood flow, temperature, skin color (from white to purple due to poor blood return via my veins), fluid accumulation (edema), and pain, even without exercise or injury. To combat the pain, I use skin patches that contain an anti-inflammatory drug, like ibuprofen or diclofenac, because the underlying problem is inflammation. Relaxation techniques such as breathing control and self-hypnosis are also quite effective, although I'm often left with some residual pain (a 2 on a scale of 0 to 10). You'll find more information about pain management in chapter 4.

The Mind Made Visible

Your mental efforts are instrumental in your physical recovery. If you're reading this book, you have what it takes to tap into the astounding power of your mind to help you get back to your life. You can't see your mind when you look in a mirror, but it's there, ready and waiting to help you on your path to recovery. The techniques and practices in this chapter will help you throughout your recovery and beyond, in the hospital and at home—which is the subject of our next chapter.

Everything You Need to Know

Your mind and your body are inextricably linked. Once you recognize that you can (and should) use your mind to help your body heal, you are heading toward a better recovery and a better quality of life. Begin a regular practice of what you've learned in this chapter and build "mental muscle" in the same way that a physical workout regimen builds stronger muscles.

- Start your gratitude journal *today*. That daily activity will nourish your resilience, sharpen your ability to focus, and strengthen your persistence.

- Develop your empathy by finding ways to show compassion for someone in need. Besides being the right thing to do, it's a habit that will replenish your energy. It will also remind you that when *you* need to ask for help, you are not burdening someone; rather, you are allowing that person to feel the reward of acting with empathy and compassion.

- Learning mindfulness will have one of the biggest impacts on your recovery. The ability to be present in the moment in a nonjudgmental state greatly improves your quality of life and your efforts in therapy. Mindfulness can be learned, but usually not simply by reading a book or watching a video. Let your health care team know that you want mindfulness training; most hospitals offer it on an outpatient basis. Or, contact a local yoga studio—they may offer mindfulness classes.

- Our understanding of neuroplasticity—the ability of the brain to create new neural pathways to restore lost function—continues to expand every day. Be sure to let your team know that you're eager to challenge yourself with functional goals that require repetition and, therefore, dedicated regular occupational and/or physical therapy.

Before You Leave the Hospital

The Five Essentials of Smart Discharge Planning

F OR THE BEST TRANSITION from the hospital to home (or wherever your next care setting may be), you need to begin formulating a plan while you are still *in* the hospital. And, because there are so many details to consider, you and your loved ones should plan as far in advance as possible. Waiting until you've left the hospital to start determining what you need isn't going to be pleasant for anyone, and the distraction won't help your rehabilitation either.

The first thing to do is to start a conversation with the doctors, nurses, and therapists caring for you in the hospital. Although it's generally hard to predict when any patient will be discharged from acute care, if your health care team knows that you and your loved ones are actively developing a plan for the next phase of your recovery, they will be more receptive to keeping the family in the loop. You'll also need their help with referrals, and the sooner your caregivers start discussing options, the better they will be able to help you and your family.

Every hospital has a department dedicated to discharge planning (also referred to as patient and family services, case management, or social work and discharge planning). This department is made up of social workers and nurses whose expertise is helping you coordinate a smooth transition from the hospital to your next destination.

A discharge planner can provide emotional support and counseling, assistance in navigating the health care system (which can save you time and money), and referrals to a multitude of diverse community resources for additional help. Local vocational rehabilitation services programs, where you can discuss your job opportunities, are excellent resources, especially if you need to change your occupation (more about this in chapter 15). In most hospitals, a discharge planner will visit you and your family within one to two days of your admission. If that doesn't happen, be sure to let your care team know you would like to meet with one.

As your discharge date gets closer, your discharge planner will return to ensure that a continuity-of-care plan is in place, including follow-up appointments with the appropriate doctors and therapists as well as any other services that you require.

In addition, every hospital has at least one officially designated patient advocate. That person can be a resource for you and your family on a wide range of issues that affect your experience as a hospitalized patient—from answering questions about medications, physical therapy, diagnosis and prognosis; palliative care options; whom on your medical team to contact for specific concerns, and so on. It's best to schedule a meeting with a patient advocate early in your hospitalization.

Hospitals are busy places. The more conversations you have with members of your team, the more comfortable you will be with the discharge process. Some people think asking questions in a hospital is an intrusion into the important work of doctors and nurses. But actually, the best health care professionals like it when patients and families speak up. It helps everyone do a better job.

The Five Essentials of Smart Discharge Planning

What I've determined, from my own experiences as a doctor and patient, and my conversations with other patients over the past ten years, is that there are five essential questions to answer as you approach the day when you will leave the hospital:

1. **When should you begin planning for discharge?** The answer is simple: as soon as possible. The process will take much longer than you might think, so try to be patient. Being hospitalized with an ANI suddenly forces you to wait for other people, and you will discover there is a real art to waiting. The first step is to lose your ego. Then, you'll need to learn to be patient, which I did by staying busy. For example, develop a stretching and exercising routine, work on dexterity by trying to pick up your medications or paper clips, or strengthen your hand muscles by squeezing a foam ball.

2. Where will you be discharged and perform rehabilitation?

There are three choices for most patients: home, a rehabilitation hospital, or a nursing home. Among the criteria that determine which will be best for you are the extent of your recovery, your medical problems and physical injuries, your ability to perform rehabilitation, the state you live in, the types of facilities near your home, and your health insurance. Your inpatient rehab team will make strong recommendations based on their knowledge of your current and future recovery, as well as their experience referring patients to specific rehab hospitals and nursing homes. In addition, for both nursing homes and in-patient rehabilitation hospitals, you should make your choice on the basis of the quality of caregivers, the ratio of therapists and nurses to patients, the number of hours that therapy is offered during the day, and statistics from the State Department of Health or national rating services such as *U.S. News & World Report* and Leapfrog Hospital Safety Grade.

There are two other key factors that should be important in your decision-making:

Continuity of care. In many hospitals, nurses work three 12-hour shifts each week and rarely see the same patient more than once or twice each week. But an excellent rehab facility will have the same two or three people assigned to you for every shift, which creates consistency that improves the safety of your care and gives them a better understanding of how to help you improve and regain function.

Choosing the facility. If possible, have your family visit the facility to determine whether it meets your personal criteria. It was important to me to choose an inpatient rehabilitation hospital that specialized in SCI. I wanted to start as soon as possible, which meant that I would be performing rehab while still on a ventilator. I also wanted to choose a highly rated hospital in a city where I would have friends and family nearby, which is how I ended up at Kessler Rehabilitation Center. Before I made my choice, my family was able to visit the facility— they liked what they saw and knew it would be a great choice for me.

- **Home:** Almost everyone wants to go home after being in the hospital. If your team believes you are ready to go home, the biggest issue will be accessibility. If you lived in an older home before your injury, the cost of remodeling to make it accessible may be prohibitive, so living in an accessible apartment while evaluating your options can be the most cost-effective approach. After my injury, my wife immediately started looking into the possibility of renovating our home, but it quickly became clear that making the house accessible would be too expensive. So she began the process of finding a place with a first-floor bedroom and bathroom. We were fortunate to find the perfect townhouse: It already had a ramp to enter the house and the wide hallways and doors that a person in a wheelchair requires. The only renovation we needed to do was to convert the existing shower to a roll-in shower. Whatever decision you make, have an occupational therapist review the areas that need to be the most accessible (bathroom, bedroom, kitchen, and entrance). They will have lots of helpful tips and suggestions on furnishings, devices, and so on, and they may also be able to suggest resources to help pay for some or all of the changes to your living space.

- **Rehabilitation facilities:** In some states, inpatient rehab facilities are freestanding hospitals. Kessler, where I was transferred after my ICU hospital stay, fits this description because the only patients there are people with SCI or TBI. Both freestanding rehabilitation hospitals and inpatient rehabilitation units in larger hospitals usually treat patients who are medically stable. For example, if you need telemetry to monitor your heart rate and rhythm, you would not qualify for this care. Some states, like New York, only permit not-for-profit hospitals, which excludes many rehabilitation hospitals. New York also doesn't allow long-term acute care hospitals, which is what most rehab hospitals are. If you live in a state that doesn't allow these types of hospitals, your options are to go to a nursing home or a long-term chronic care facility, such as a county hospital, or to travel to a hospital out of state.

- **Nursing homes:** If you are severely injured, you will likely be discharged from the hospital to a nursing home, because the seriousness of your injuries prevents you from engaging in rigorous rehab. If you have a medical problem, such as heart failure or a pressure ulcer that makes you a poor candidate for intensive rehabilitation, you may also go to a nursing home. Some nursing homes have special rehabilitation units that include physiatrists, occupational and physical therapists, and speech and language pathologists. In states that don't have freestanding rehab hospitals, the only choice for people on Medicaid is to go to a nursing home for long-term recovery.

3. **Who will take care of you after you are discharged?**
Contemporary rehab care requires an entire team of health providers working together. When you are in the hospital ICU, the physician specializing in your care is usually a trauma specialist or neurologist. A change in your attending physician usually occurs when you are transferred to a specialized rehab unit. The rehabilitation physician is usually a physiatrist who has completed a residency in physical medicine and rehabilitation (PM&R). They are responsible for treating medical issues, formulating therapeutic goals, interacting with your other health care providers, and discussing your progress with you and your loved ones.

The other members of the team usually include nurses and aides; therapists with expertise in physical, occupational, speech, and recreational therapy, as well as vocational rehab; psychologists; social workers; and a case manager. Additional team members may include a driving instructor, peer mentor, nutritionist, and equipment specialist. Every member of your health care team should consider your family additional team members.

If you are discharged to your home, you may need referrals to specialists in addition to your primary care physician (PCP), because you may need to see a physiatrist, a neurologist, a pain specialist, and possibly a urologist and a gastroenterologist. You may not be able to find doctors with specialized training, but it is worth inquiring while you're still in the hospital. You will also need a referral from your PCP or physiatrist for physical and occupational therapy. Your doctor will likely recommend an ambulatory rehab facility near your home, but you should spend time interviewing some of their therapists to determine that the facility has well-trained clinicians with expertise in your particular injury.

Once you are discharged from the hospital, you will be responsible for many aspects of your own care. At home, someone needs to help you attend to the everyday issues of personal hygiene, pain treatment, medications (especially the side effects), sleep, nutrition, rehabilitation therapy, and exercise. Have the hospital's discharge planner identify the social workers in your community with the right expertise, and the home care and rehabilitation options that you'll need. Depending on your situation, these may include someone to drive you to and from work and to appointments with your doctors, therapists, and other health care providers (acupuncture, exercise classes, massage, nutritionist, and so on). With the help of your discharge planner, you can learn what services are available in your community, how to get them, and how to pay for them. While your health insurance will be the primary source of money to pay for these expenses, a social worker and case manager will be important to help you identify other ways to pay for your needs, such as workers' compensation, Medicare, Medicaid, and vocational rehabilitation.

You may also want to consider hiring a home aide. A week before I was discharged, I interviewed several home aides recommended by friends, medical colleagues, and social workers. I was fortunate to find a certified home health aide who had previous experience working with paralyzed individuals. The industry standard for certification programs in home health is 120 hours of classroom training and 40 to 60 hours of clinical work. She stayed with me in the hospital from morning to night for several days to learn my routine from the nurses and aides. She learned how to transfer me in and out of my bed and wheelchair, get me dressed, change my night and day urine collection bags, and help me in the bathroom.

4. **What types of durable medical equipment (DME) will you need to purchase or rent?** While you are in the hospital, you and your team will figure out what DME you'll need after you leave the hospital. Social Security defines DME as equipment that can withstand repeated use, is used primarily to serve a medical purpose, and is appropriate for use in the home.

Nothing is more important than choosing the right wheelchair, because you will spend most of your day in it, and you'll need it to last for at least

Choosing Equipment for Discharge

Because I was a tetraplegic, I had to choose an electric wheelchair while I was in rehab, because they are manufactured to individual specifications and some of them are made overseas. My rehab facility had several different models to test. After two weeks of testing six models, I decided to purchase the Permobil wheelchair, because it was easy to drive in a straight line and it fit me well. Because these wheelchairs are made in Sweden, mine didn't arrive for six weeks after I placed the order. That meant I needed to rent a wheelchair for at least a month. For my health insurance to pay for both the permanent chair and the loaner, my doctors and therapists needed to justify why the Permobil chair was the one I needed and write a prescription. This may be the case for you, too.

Most patients don't have the equipment necessary for them to function well at home. I certainly didn't. I needed to purchase a hospital bed, a shower chair that could also be positioned over the toilet, a commode, and a Hoyer lift to move me from my bed to my wheelchair. To make decisions about my DME, I was assisted by my physical therapist and a local sales representative whose company specialized in DME.

five years. The critical issues in choosing an electric wheelchair to consider are ease of controls, the ability to tilt the chair for pressure relief, the nature of the driving mechanism (so that you can be confident going up and down steep inclines and through tight doorways), whether it can change your height off the ground for social occasions, and so on (see chapter 15 for an in-depth wheelchair guide). It can take several weeks for a customized wheelchair to be delivered, so you should begin the process of purchasing one at least one month before discharge. For a push wheelchair, the options are fewer, but the process is very similar. You must test the chair to make sure it fits you well, that the foot rest is comfortable, the chair is light enough to make it easy to push but sturdy enough to be stable for transfers, and that folding and storage are easy to perform.

For transportation to medical appointments, your job, social events—whatever the need may be—you might require a special vehicle. The design of the vehicle (often a van) will depend on your physical abilities, especially your hand and arm function. Most people with an ANI will be able to drive using normal cars fitted with adaptive hand controls. These can be as simple as a device that makes it easier to turn the wheel, or as complex as $40,000 hand controls that help you use the brakes, gas pedal, signals, mirrors, wipers, and radio. If you have severe disabilities and are in an electric wheelchair that weighs at least 300 pounds, a van will be necessary so that you can enter and exit the vehicle via a ramp. If you are moderately disabled (especially if your upper arm strength is weak, making transfers difficult), you may prefer a driver's seat that rotates to facilitate transfer from your wheelchair to the driver's seat. In my case, driving is too much of a mental and physical effort to make it worthwhile, so I arrange for a driver to take me to my appointments. While that can be inconvenient at times, safety is always my first priority.

After an ANI, you will be introduced to the world of assistive devices. You've probably already used many of these without even thinking about it, such as a TV remote. The most important assistive device I used in the hospital was my laptop computer with Dragon Dictation Software that I used to answer emails. When I returned to work, I wanted to start using all of the programs I had used pre-injury, such as Microsoft Office, but I found that my computer's touchpad and mouse were too difficult for me to manipulate. Because there are so many computer manufacturers and even more types of mice, it will be helpful for you to experiment with several options.

The perfect solution for me appeared in April 2010, when the first iPad was introduced. With the iPad, I could perform many functions just by gently moving my finger, which was good for my physical therapy and gave me greater independence. Now, there are numerous handheld devices and apps. You'll find a list of them in the Resources on page 283. If you can't afford to pay for them, your employer may be able to; make sure to check with your social worker and your health insurance company.

5. **Why does it take so much time to figure out how to pay for everything?** There are two reasons why paying the bills after an ANI takes so much time. First, it's very expensive, so you will usually need more than one insurance product. Second, there are many insurance forms to fill out, especially if you have specialized medical or physical disabilities. For many people, an ANI is not only a catastrophic physical event but also a financial one. Depending on the nature of the injury, costs can exceed $100,000 in the first year. So it's important that you have health insurance to help you pay for these costs.

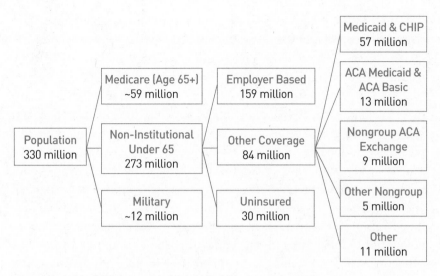

Figure 11. US healthcare coverage: ACA (Affordable Care Act), CHIP

There are four public insurance plans that cover about 40 percent of US citizens: Medicare, Military, Medicaid, and Children's Health Insurance Program (CHIP). Nongovernment insurance includes employer-based insurance, which includes about 48 percent of US citizens. The remaining 12 percent are either uninsured or have other types of insurance as indicated.

As soon as possible after you are admitted to the hospital, you and your family should work with your social worker to assess your health insurance plan. If you qualify for public insurance, a social worker can help you apply. If you are over sixty-five, you and your social worker should work to determine your eligibility for Medicaid or Medicare. If you have employer-based insurance, ask your employer's human resources representative to work with you and your insurer. You will likely be assigned a case manager from the insurance company to work with you, your family, and the hospital to facilitate your care in the hospital and plan for your care after discharge. This person is also called a designated claims adviser or benefits provider. They must clearly understand your therapy needs, because they will be your advocate when it comes to using your benefits and getting the most coverage out of your plan. A good case manager will want to know your previous health history, learn the risk factors you have for secondary complications and arrange for preventive therapy, and understand the necessary treatments you need to maintain your health. This kind of approach with your insurance company is a win-win—you obtain the services you need and the insurance company spends less money on acute care because you will be less likely to be readmitted to the hospital.

If your injury is severe and you're unable to return to work, you have three options. First, if you were employed at the time of your accident, you may have disability insurance that begins one to three months after you stop working and pays you 50 to 75 percent of your salary. This is the time to notify that insurance company of the need to file a claim. Second, if you do not have disability insurance and you are permanently disabled, you should sign up for Medicaid Social Security Disability Insurance (SSDI). SSDI payments are made on the basis of financial need. SSDI does not pay for hospital care directly; rather, it enables you to pay for essential expenses such as your mortgage, gas and electric, prescription drugs, and vocational rehabilitation. The process of obtaining SSDI, Medicaid, or Medicare is *slow*, so start the applications as soon as you've evaluated your financial resources and expenses. Third, take a look at your life insurance policy; if it's a whole life policy, you should be able to take money from it to use for current health expenditures. While this will reduce the final value of the policy, it can provide necessary money if you need it.

If you have no insurance, the hospital will assign a social worker to help you apply for Medicaid (if you qualify), purchase insurance on the health exchange (if you can afford it), or work with you on a payment plan that may include charity care (in which case some of your charges will be paid by the hospital). You will have a lot going on, and it may be difficult for you to remember everything, so be sure that someone on your team takes notes and keeps a record of all of these meetings.

Navigating the health insurance system can be difficult. Your case manager can confirm what your insurance policy pays for, what it doesn't, what portion is a copay that you are responsible for, and so on. Communicating with your insurance provider can be tricky, so be prepared to spend hours on the phone, if necessary. The good news is that you can have the social worker in charge of your continuity of care initiate meetings with your insurance company's case manager, with a family member acting as your advocate. Your social worker will be able to ensure that you have the coverage you need, and a good case manager will work hard to get you the best care for the lowest cost.

Whatever kind of health and/or disability insurance plan you have at the time of your injury, your social worker will want to obtain a copy of it to review the full explanation of your insurance benefits (EOB). Your social worker should also set up a meeting in which you, the social worker/discharge planner, and the insurance company's case manager review the EOB. To prepare for this meeting, ask the doctor overseeing your care in the hospital to refer you to the outpatient services you will need after discharge, such as physical therapy and speech therapy. Your doctor's written referral is required for your insurance plan to pay for care, whether partially or in full. This means not only that the insurance company has what it needs to process the claim but that the therapist can provide feedback to the physiatrist to update the therapy prescription as needed. Have a family member or aide at that meeting to take notes and to highlight relevant sections of the EOB. Record every interaction with your insurance company and date it. It can also help to have a large envelope where you can keep copies of prescriptions for therapy, medicine, and devices, as well as any bills you receive for co- or full payment for any of those items.

If you are being discharged to a rehab hospital or a nursing home, you'll want to know how many days of coverage are allowed for inpatient hospitalization, and if you can go directly home, the coverage for ambulatory and home health rehabilitation. Find out if your policy allows you to use a facility that is out of state, because there may be a better out-of-state facility that specializes in your injury. If you can, find out the maximum number of days allowed in the rehab facility and if there is a lifetime cap on the number of days allowed in each care facility.

Your social worker will also look at what your insurance allows regarding your choice of hospitals and doctors. Many hospitals are part of larger networks that encompass broad geographical areas. Within these networks, there's usually one large hospital that handles the most serious patients. For example, my accident happened less than ten miles from the F. F. Thompson Hospital in Canandaigua, but because I needed a Level 1 Trauma Center, I was airlifted to the largest hospital in the area, Strong Memorial Hospital, in Rochester, forty-five miles away. This hospital has specialized personnel, equipment, and facilities to treat Level 1 trauma patients (which often includes SCI and TBI patients) and is a comprehensive stroke center.

It's not unusual to hear that dealing with the insurance company is hard work, but your primary focus should be on recovery and rehabilitation, not on the ins and out of your insurance plan. Reach out to the members of your health care team who are experts at navigating health insurance, and let them lift the burden so you can put your energy into healing and recovery.

Once you are ready for discharge, your next challenges will be to continue your functional recovery, maintain your health, and work on changes in your lifestyle that promote wellness.

––––––

Everything You Need to Know

Discharge from the hospital is an exciting prospect, but it's one that requires planning with as much lead time as possible. Begin discussing the options with your hospital health care team as soon as possible. Whether the next phase of recovery results in discharge to a rehabilitation hospital, a nursing home, or your own home, you'll need to consider the five Ws of smart discharge planning: When, Where, Who, What, and Why:

- **When:** When should you begin planning for discharge? Even though your initial focus will be on simply getting out of the hospital, don't wait until then to start making arrangements for the transition. You and your family should begin these discussions with your physician and therapists as early as possible.

- **Where:** Where will you live once discharged from the hospital? Is your home set up for your current physical disabilities? If you go to a nursing home, and if you're able to choose it, ask your physician for a recommendation. If your insurance allows you to go to a specialized rehabilitation hospital before going home, consider the advantages, even if the facility is out of state.

- **Who:** Who will care for you when you are discharged? Who will oversee that care? If you will be discharged to your home, your loved ones will need to ensure that home care arrangements are in place, as well as outpatient therapies. You may also need to get referrals to medical specialists if your only doctor is a primary care physician. Ask for those referrals while you are still in the hospital.

- **What:** What types of medical equipment will you need after you leave the hospital? A wheelchair? Ramp? Specially equipped car? Work with your therapy team to make those decisions, and work with the social worker and case manager to determine how they will be paid for.

- **Why:** As you face the exciting yet nerve-wracking prospect of finally being discharged from the hospital, you will be entering a new phase of recovery that can be difficult physically, mentally, and emotionally. The fact that this is the time that you have to arrange for health care coverage and insurance is an unfortunate consequence of the US health care system. It's best to work closely with your social worker (and case manager, if you have one) to choose which insurance coverage and insurance plan are best for you. If you find yourself asking, *Why am I putting myself through this?*, remember what you have to gain—for yourself, your family, and for other people with disabilities who will look to you for inspiration.

PART 2

Functional Recovery, Health, and Wellness

Pain Management

Controlling Pain Helps Speed Your Rehabilitation

W HAT EXACTLY IS PAIN? The International Association for the Study
of Pain defines it as "an unpleasant sensory and emotional experience associated with, or resembling that associated with, actual or potential
tissue damage."[1] Pain is complex; it includes an *emotional* component that
affects thinking and behavior, as well as a *physical* component that limits
movement and function.

Each person experiences pain differently, so your pain may differ significantly from that of someone with a similar injury. Determining how
your pain is produced and experienced will guide the choices for the best
treatment approaches for you. A multidisciplinary approach is best. This
can include drugs; application of heat and cold; the use of ultrasound;
cognitive and behavioral therapies; complementary medicine (acupuncture, cannabis, meditation, hypnosis, biofeedback, yoga, massage); exercise;
devices such as transcutaneous electrical nerve stimulation (TENS); epidural electrical stimulation; and intrathecal drug delivery (injecting medications directly into the spinal canal that surrounds the spinal cord). I
recommend combining therapies that provide synergistic pain relief with
minimal side effects. Avoid narcotics, if possible (or work with your doctor to wean yourself off them as soon as possible), because they are highly
addictive and can have harmful long-term effects on your ability to perform rehabilitation and return to work.

The nature of your pain (sharp versus dull, or burning versus freezing,
for example) is not nearly as important as the *frequency and duration*. I have
felt some kind of pain every day for the last eleven years, which means my
pain is chronic. On a scale of 0 to 10, it varies from a 1 to an 8, depending
on a multitude of factors, including stress, medications, exercise, urinary

tract infections, among others. As you no doubt already know, pain will sap your energy, limit your sleep, make you irritable and prone to anger, and limit your rehabilitation, so I've found ways to address mine. My tactics have evolved over the years, and what works for me may not suit you, but "grinning and bearing it" is really not an option. That's no way to live your life, which is why *effective treatment of pain is a necessity*. As you begin your pain management journey, don't expect any single treatment to completely *eliminate* your pain; keep in mind that pain management is successful even if it only reduces the severity of pain. But this shift can make an enormous difference!

My Pain Journey

My own battle with pain began in the hospital, right after my accident. Even though I was paralyzed, I felt pain everywhere, coming in waves that overwhelmed my ability to think. It's likely that the pain was caused by the surgery I had undergone, combined with the pain of being intubated. Mercifully, the doctors had ordered an excellent painkiller, Dilaudid (hydromorphone), a derivative of morphine. Within a minute of receiving it, I would be transported to a state of bliss; I felt like I was floating in space and was completely without pain. Unfortunately, Dilaudid could not be my long-term pain medicine because it's almost always given intravenously, it's highly addictive, and it causes constipation.

One hundred and twelve days later, when I was discharged from Kessler Rehabilitation Center to return for further inpatient rehabilitation in Rochester, my pain medicine of choice had become Vicodin, another opiate (specifically, a combination of hydrocodone and acetaminophen). Before I got into the van, I took two Vicodin. I needed another four hours later; the roads were bumpy, which made my shoulders hurt terribly. But as my wife pulled into the admissions bay at Strong Memorial Hospital, I was flooded with emotion to finally be home, back in my city (and at my hospital). Filled with elation, I promised myself I would never take opiate drugs again. Those drugs had addressed my pain well, but the side effects (fuzzy mind, constipation) were not things I wanted to live with for the long term.

I wasn't able to keep that promise to myself, at least not immediately; it was still too early in my recovery. After every physical therapy session, the pain in my shoulders was so great that nonsteroidal anti-inflammatory drugs (NSAIDs) were not sufficient to reduce it. Instead, I was given a fentanyl patch, which was adjusted by slowly increasing the dose until it brought my pain level down to a 1. Over the next month, my pain became more localized, in my right upper chest and biceps. This was both musculoskeletal and neuropathic pain. The musculoskeletal pain was caused by ambulating with my platform walker, which required me to support myself with my forearms. The neuropathic pain was a burning sensation when I touched my skin. So I began using a topical patch that released lidocaine (Lidoderm) locally to numb the pain.

By the time I left Strong Memorial Hospital's rehab unit on October 7, 2009 (four months after my accident), my pain medications included:

- Duragesic (fentanyl patch) for generalized severe pain
- Lyrica (pregabalin), 150 mg, three times per day for neuropathic pain
- Lidoderm (lidocaine) patches, a fast-acting local anesthetic
- Flector (diclofenac) patches, an anti-inflammatory pain reliever for musculoskeletal pain
- Zanaflex (tizanidine), a muscle relaxant that decreases tightness and spasticity everywhere, thereby decreasing pain

That's quite a list of powerful drugs, but they made it possible for me to work hard on my physical and occupational therapies, to be with my loved ones without being distracted by debilitating pain, and to be able to concentrate, think, and, eventually, return to work.

Acute versus Chronic Pain

Pain can be characterized as acute or chronic. You may frequently experience both. **Acute pain,** like the pain you feel when you burn yourself on the stove, are stung by a bee, or break a bone, is a *physiologic response* that alerts you to the injury. This involuntary reaction is part of our survival mechanism. While the pain of a broken bone is more intense and lasts longer than that of a bee sting, the pain diminishes and then disappears within a pretty predictable time frame in both situations—two days for a bee sting, and two months to a year for a broken bone. **Chronic pain,** in contrast, lasts beyond a "typical" time frame and is frequently part of a complex biopsychosocial situation in which emotions, environment, and social interactions play significant roles in generating pain.

Nociceptive versus Neuropathic Pain

Pain can be divided into two categories based on the process by which it arises. Nociceptive pain comes from damaged tissue and nerve fibers, such as that caused by cutting your hand while using a knife. It feels burning, stabbing, or throbbing, and usually gets significantly better within hours to days. In contrast, neuropathic pain comes from damage to the nervous system *itself*. Specifically, the peripheral and central nervous system (called the somatosensory system) are damaged by nerve trauma or nerve diseases. Neuropathic pain also differs from nociceptive pain because it is more likely to be chronic, with months to years without improvement. It can cause you to feel abnormal nerve sensations called dysesthesias and paresthesias, which are usually felt in the arms, hands, legs, or feet. Paresthesia and dysesthesia differ in severity. Paresthesia is more sensation than pain, a tingling or pins-and-needles feeling. Dysesthesia is usually painful; it frequently causes a burning sensation, and it's not explained by an obvious injury to a limb but may be "created" centrally in your brain. Finally, allodynia is hypersensitivity—it describes pain from a stimulus, such as light touch, that is not normally painful.

Neuropathic pain is especially common after ANI. It's the kind of pain that's "all in your head," because it really is self-created, at least in part. Consequently, the nature of the pain sensation, the situations that cause the pain, and what makes it better or worse are unique to each individual. Neuropathic pain can originate from anywhere in the body where there are nerves: in the sensory nerves in your skin, nerves in your spine, and nerves in the brain itself. The most widely known example of neuropathic pain is phantom limb pain, which is when you feel pain from a limb that is no longer present. In this case, damage to the nerves of that limb causes a reorganization (a kind of neuroplasticity) of the transmission, modulation, and perception of pain by the brain.

My Neuropathic Pain

I have three types of neuropathic pain. My right upper chest is exquisitely sensitive to touch (allodynia), which can elicit a burning sensation. My right bicep gets very tight, resulting in a dull, throbbing, steady pain (dysesthesia). I usually wake up around 4:00 AM because my forearms and hands feel like they are encased in concrete (paresthesia). I know that all of these pains occur because my brain is not receiving sensory input from my muscles and nerves because so many nerves were killed by my SCI. Even so, it's still debilitating. The good news is that it's treatable.

Spasticity

Spasticity is a side effect of paralysis that increases muscle tone (tightness). It's caused when there is damage to the parts of the brain or spinal cord that control voluntary movements, and the symptoms range from stiffness to uncontrolled spasms. Spasticity can cause severe pain, or it may have no effect on your daily life. My spasticity causes my right upper arm to tighten progressively over the course of the day, causing increased pain. It can make one of my legs get stuck behind the other when I try to walk. Spasticity can limit your range of motion, and thereby your independence. It also increases with other health problems, such as constipation or urinary tract infections.

Paying attention to spasticity is important. There are several effective drugs for spasticity, including baclofen, tizanidine, and clonazepam. They all have side effects, so try several to find the one that works best for you. Regular stretching to maintain flexibility and using hot packs or a vibrating massage device can reduce spasticity significantly. If you have severe spasticity, especially with pain, talk to your doctor about the option of having a small pump implanted that infuses baclofen directly into your spinal canal. Since the pump contains a lower dosage than oral medication, the side effects are minimized.

Pain Treatment and Management

Controlling your pain is essential to your recovery. Don't tough it out. Managing your pain with prescription and over-the-counter drugs, as well as non-drug therapies, will help you tamp down pain so that you can work on your rehabilitation. Your goal, as you try different treatments, is to find approaches that reduce your pain with few or no side effects and few or no interactions with other drugs. As you will learn, there's usually no single drug that possesses all these properties.

You should also seek to optimize treatment of *other* conditions that might sensitize your perception of pain. Treatment of high blood pressure, heart failure, diabetes, and other medical problems should be handled *before* you start drug treatment for pain. This is particularly true if you have muscle spasticity and increased tightness (tone); treatments to reduce muscle tightness (such as baclofen and tizanidine) will dramatically lessen the need for pain treatment.

Drug Therapies

Drugs can be an essential part of pain management as you embark on rehabilitation, but long-term use of drugs should be avoided as much as possible, because all drugs have side effects that may become harmful over time, and different drugs may interact with each other to create new side effects. Drugs should always be used in conjunction with nonpharmacologic approaches, which we'll explore later in this chapter. For many patients, using combinations of drugs that target different metabolic and nerve pathways can result in improved pain relief and fewer side effects, because this allows for lower doses of each drug. Combination therapy is often necessary because fewer than half of individuals with neuropathic pain respond to a single drug.[2]

Medications should be administered through the most effective and comfortable route, allowing you the maximum amount of control. Pain relievers for moderate to severe pain should be taken on a fixed dose and scheduled around the clock and not on an "as needed" basis. This approach will allow for more consistent pain relief, since you don't have to play catch-up after a previous dose has worn off.

For neuropathic pain, the most common drugs are ones also used to treat other conditions.[3] These can be medicines that prevent depression (tricyclic antidepressants such as amitriptyline or nortriptyline), because they decrease activation of brain areas that process pain. Chronic pain can cause depression, and vice versa, setting in place a vicious cycle. Drugs that prevent seizures (anti-epileptics, such as gabapentin or pregabalin) are also effective for pain relief, because they calm hyperactive nerves. Serotonin norepinephrine uptake inhibitors (SNRIs such as venlafaxine (Effexor) and duloxetine (Cymbalta) have been used as initial treatment because of fewer side effects than tricyclic antidepressants. Opioids are third-line drugs due to the risk of dependency, addiction, and overdose.

The pharmacologic approach to nociceptive pain primarily involves nonsteroidal anti-inflammatory drugs (NSAIDs), such as ibuprofen (Advil), diclofenac (Voltaren), and naproxen (Aleve, Naprosyn).

Cannabis and cannabinoids: Cannabis (marijuana) has been used for thousands of years to treat pain and enjoy a state of relaxation. There are two widely available species (types) of cannabis: Indica and Sativa. There's a common misunderstanding that Sativa energizes you and Indica relaxes you. But the truth is that almost all cannabis comes from hybrids of these two species, because hybrid plants grow larger and faster, and they're more resistant to disease. The cannabis plant contains cannabinoids, which are compounds that bind to specific receptors in the brain, spinal cord, and other organs. The best-known cannabinoid is tetrahydrocannabinol (THC), which is responsible for most of the psychoactive effects, including relaxation, euphoria, and hunger. The other important cannabinoid is cannabidiol (CBD).

To understand the use of cannabis for treatment of pain, we must first start with definitions of the preparations that are available for use. "Medical marijuana" is dried material from the cannabis plant, consisting of THC, CBD, and other cannabinoids. Medical marijuana can be purchased from dispensaries in a variety of preparations. Some dispensaries sell medical marijuana that has been grown under conditions (type of seeds, hydroponics versus soil, UV light versus sunlight versus special colors) that increase the amount of CBD relative to THC. It's not sold in pharmacies, because it's not legal at the federal level, only on a state-by-state basis, and it's not currently available for insurance coverage. However, when properly cultivated and analyzed for relative concentrations of CBD and THC, the medical marijuana sold in the dispensaries may be safer than marijuana purchased in "retail settings."

The FDA has approved one cannabis-derived drug product: Epidiolex (CBD), and three synthetic cannabis–related drug products: Marinol (dronabinol), Syndros (dronabinol), and Cesamet (nabilone).[4] These approved drugs are available with a prescription from a licensed health care provider (usually with special training for Schedule I drugs, which include cannabis). These cannabinoids are FDA-approved for the treatment of pediatric epilepsies, chemotherapy–induced nausea and vomiting, and extreme weight-loss conditions, like AIDS. All other medical conditions will be "off-label," and therefore not covered by insurance.

The data in the medical literature on the use of cannabis for chronic pain treatment is equivocal but overall negative. But many of the studies did not use well-defined cannabis preparations. The best studies used the FDA-approved cannabinoids (dronabinol and nabilone), which lack THC and therefore have fewer euphoric effects and almost no physical effects. A survey of ninety-one publications that used CBD showed no benefit compared to placebo for chronic pain.[5] More than half of the people studied had neuropathic pain; they also showed no benefit. However, there was a large increase in harmful effects related to mental, physical, and emotional function among study participants who received CBD. A 2017 meta-analysis of twenty-seven studies examining the effectiveness of cannabis in treating chronic pain found only weak evidence that cannabis alleviated neuropathic pain, and no evidence suggesting that cannabis was useful in other types of pain.[6] Overall, the careful randomized studies of cannabis-based medicine (herbal cannabis, plant-derived or synthetic THC, THC/CBD nasal spray) in chronic neuropathic pain show that the potential benefit may be less than their potential harm.

There are two factors, in my opinion, that affect the efficacy of cannabis-derived products as treatment for neuropathic pain. The first is the method of ingestion, and the second is the relative amount of THC versus CBD. There are several small randomized trials that show short-term benefit for smoked[7] or vaporized cannabis[8] in patients with neuropathic pain. Unfortunately, these small studies did not report the amount of THC versus CBD, and there were side effects that caused about 20 percent of the patients to stop their use.

If you choose to include cannabis as part of your pain relief regimen, it's important to use medical cannabis distributed by a pharmacy or dispensary, because cannabis grown for recreational use isn't suitable for medical use. It's not FDA-approved, nor is its composition and potency regulated, so it's not possible to predict its efficacy and side effects from one purchase to the next. It's also important to note that when you smoke cannabis for medical use, you will be exposed to all the dangers associated with smoking cigarettes, including the possibility that the cannabis may contain contaminants, which can damage your lungs. It also has the potential to become addictive, causing increased tolerance and withdrawal symptoms that make it difficult to stop. Furthermore, the physiologic effects of smoked or vaped THC may negatively affect your ability to function in work or school.

Therefore, medical marijuana should only be used when other treatments for neuropathic pain have not helped. If this applies to you, work with your doctor and dispensary pharmacist to find the dosage, relative amounts of THC versus other cannabinoids in the preparation, and the type of delivery (oil by mouth, edible, or topical) of medical cannabis that are effective and safe for you. Note that dispensaries do not sell preparations that can be smoked or vaped.

Lidocaine infusion: Lidocaine is often used for local anesthesia, to numb the nerves that cause nociceptive pain, before surgical (often dental) procedures. But several studies have shown that it can also be useful in treating chronic neuropathic pain. In outpatient settings, doses of 3 to 5 mg/kg administered over 30 to 60 minutes can relieve neuropathic pain in the short term, with sustained benefit of several months in about 40 percent of patients.[9]

Topical therapies: There are three widely available drugs you can use on your skin for local pain relief without systemic side effects. All three use a gel pad in which the drug slowly passes from the gel into your skin providing 8 to 12 hours of pain relief. The lidocaine (Lidoderm) patch is most effective in treating allodynia. The diclofenac (Flector) patch is the most common of several NSAIDs that exist in patch form. While it is best used for acute muscle and joint pain, it has also been useful in patients with neuropathic pain that is caused by inflammation such as complex regional pain syndrome (CRPS). Capsaicin is a compound derived from chili peppers that is thought to decrease pain by inhibiting pain-sensing nerves in the skin. It is most commonly used in creams, which must be applied every 6 to 8 hours for several weeks to achieve maximum benefit. I found it useful for my right chest pain, but after a couple of months of use, I developed burning and a red allergic rash (this occurs in about 40 percent of patients), so I had to stop using it.

Decreasing Your Dosage

Over time and as appropriate, you should try to decrease your drug intake. Why? Because taking as few drugs as possible means decreasing unwanted side effects, which will improve your quality of life. Here are my guidelines to help you get there:

- Only make changes to your medications based on consultation with your doctor. That person can be your primary care physician, your physiatrist, or another pain specialist. In most situations, it's up to you to initiate a decrease in medications. If you don't say anything, your doctor will think that everything is OK. In response to your request, they will likely try to decrease your dose by 50 percent over the course of three months. If you're fortunate, you will eventually find that you're able to completely stop taking a medicine or that you can take it at a greatly reduced dose.

- Begin with the medicine that is causing the most side effects, especially those that affect your thinking, bowels, libido, sleep, or energy.

- Stop medications that work through the same mechanism. For example, oxycontin and fentanyl are both opiates, so you should not be taking them at the same time. Sometimes, two doctors will start you on different medications for the same problem, especially if your list of prescribed drugs is not updated. This can easily occur when your doctor is not using an electronic medical record (EMR), or their EMR is different from the next doctor that you see. Make sure that you bring a current list with you to your appointment, and that your doctor reviews your medication list. Use drugs that are synergistic; one drug should enhance the actions of another.

- Keep in mind that drug titration (slowly increasing or decreasing the dose of a medication until you find the right balance between positive effects and negative side effects) is part of achieving pain relief. It can take a while to arrive at the correct combination of drugs and doses, so don't lose faith if it sometimes feels like you're taking two steps forward and one step back.

In the eleven years since my injury, I've been able to wean off a *lot* of drugs or have greatly decreased the dosage. I found that a combination of exercise and massage—and paying attention to actions that caused muscle pain—allowed me to gradually discontinue my fentanyl patch in three months. Within six months, I was able to achieve pain control using Lyrica, Flector, and Tylenol instead. Drug titration is an ongoing process—so don't get discouraged if it takes a while to figure out what works best for you.

Behavioral Approaches to Pain Management

When developing a pain management routine, don't limit yourself to just medication. Be open to nonpharmaceutical approaches to reduce pain, such as exercise, acupuncture, massage, meditation, and yoga (see chapter 8 for more information). I found these therapies beneficial during my rehab and continue to use them to this day. As you consider these options, keep in mind that the skills and techniques of therapists can vary widely. If the first one you try doesn't help, that doesn't mean that the *technique* is not useful; it could be that therapist isn't suited to your needs.

Exercise

Exercise can be one of the most helpful therapies for pain. It works by stimulating the modulating nerves that inhibit transmission of pain and by raising the threshold for pain. Exercise also requires concentration, which can distract you from pain. The benefits are mental as well as physical, because your brain releases endorphins (the "runner's high") that make you feel good. Talk with your therapists about an exercise routine that will improve your cardiovascular fitness. This increases blood supply, improving your endurance so that muscle fatigue and pain occur only after extended use. The increase in strength makes it less likely that you will sustain an overuse injury, which would cause nociceptive pain that can trigger neuropathic pain. I try to do some form of cardiovascular exercise, usually stationary cycling, for forty-five minutes every day. I also perform more focused occupational or physical therapy, or weight-lifting, for thirty minutes every other day. I've found that using my entire body for exercise helps decrease the localized pain in my right arm.

Cognitive behavioral therapy (CBT) uses your own thought processes to help you gain control over your pain.[10] It works in two ways: First, it activates the modulating pathways that descend from the brain to inhibit transmission of pain; and second, it teaches you how to control your pain rather than be controlled by it. CBT techniques include relaxation, physical exercise, imagery, desensitization exercises, and goal setting, to train yourself to develop the ability to handle pain. Training yourself to separate your emotions from your pain allows you to work through it and thereby function better. Used in conjunction with other pain-relief therapies, CBT can be an important component of your long-term pain management program. (For more on CBT, see page 22.)

Relaxation techniques can help diminish chronic pain by inhibiting pain transmission from the brain. These techniques include meditation (see page 79), learned deep relaxation, guided imagery, self-hypnosis, and mindfulness. In each of these approaches, you learn how to focus your mind and prevent intruding thoughts and external stimuli from distracting you. These approaches work by decreasing sympathetic nervous system (SNS) activity (the fight-or-flight axis). Among them, meditation and mindfulness can be very helpful, but you may need to work with your therapy team to find the ones that feel most comfortable for you. These techniques are noninvasive, do not require drugs, and can be performed at home. Personally, I use a combination of yoga breathing, self-hypnosis, and meditation.

Thermotherapy, Ultrasound, Hydrotherapy, and Cryotherapy

Thermotherapy is heat therapy used to improve blood flow to muscles that have become painful due to overuse. Too much activity (as can easily occur with paralyzed muscles during exercise) builds up lactic acid, which is painful. Heat opens the blood vessels to the affected area and speeds removal of the lactic acid. Muscle spasms can also respond to heat, particularly if they form a knot, like a charley horse. There are many ways to use therapeutic heat. Moist heat and a heavy material that keeps it in place seem to be the best from my personal experience, as does a warm shower or hot bath. Heating pads work well, as do the more expensive heated massage pads that can be purchased from specialty stores. One warning: When applying heat to body parts with diminished sensation, make sure to have someone else check the temperature or place it against a part of your body that senses temperature well, like your face, so that you don't experience a burn.

Ultrasound is a noninvasive way to obtain images of internal organs such as the bladder, heart, and kidney. But it can also be used to provide relief from both pain and muscle spasms, by heating deep tissues with sound waves, which penetrate farther than topical heat, to warm tendons, ligaments, and fascia. Phonophoresis is the use of ultrasound to deliver topically applied pain-relieving drugs to the tissues. I recommend trying ultrasound first, because there is much debate over whether phonophoresis is any better than high-frequency ultrasound alone. If you don't notice improvement after three treatments, ultrasound is unlikely to be helpful for you. This may be because the inflamed tissue is too deep for the ultrasound to penetrate or that the problem is not inflammation.

Hydrotherapy is like a whirlpool bath, which involves placing the painful limb in swirling warm water for fifteen to thirty minutes. It works similarly to ultrasound treatment in terms of warming the affected limb. I found it very useful for my feet, which are hard to treat with ultrasound.

Cryotherapy, the application of cold, can be effective at decreasing nerve and muscle pain. Cold slows the speed of nerve transmission, making it harder for pain signals to reach the brain. It also decreases muscle spasms, which contribute significantly to pain perception. And, if exercise has damaged muscle, cold will decrease the inflammation. For best results, apply cold every one to two hours, for twenty minutes at a time. I like to use flexible ice packs with Velcro tabs that hold them in place.

Massage, Acupuncture, Trigger Point Therapy, Myofascial Release, and Other Therapies

These therapies can be very useful when used in conjunction with other methods of pain control.[11] All four techniques treat sites where muscles, nerves, and myofascia combine to form small knots, also called trigger points. These sites are frequently associated with increased spasticity and tone that pinch off the blood supply and cause pain. The myofascia, a thick layer of fibrous material that surrounds muscle bundles, normally stretches like a rubber band, allowing nerves and blood vessels to slide between the bundles. After injury or prolonged immobilization, the fascia can stiffen and become inflamed, making it less flexible. This change can "trap" the nerves, further irritating them and causing pain with movement. The fascia also has sensory receptors that can transmit pain. In rare situations, injections of lidocaine and steroids may be helpful. A number of therapists incorporate the concept of trigger points and myofascial disease into a therapeutic massage modality (see more in chapter 8). The long-term benefits of myofascial release remain to be proven, so it should not be a primary therapy for pain management.

- **Acupuncture:** Some acupuncturists treat local pain by using needles to target dysfunctional muscles and joints, but many use a broader concept of organ and tissue health that can't be manipulated by stimulating specific points. The broader approach focuses on increasing your qi (vital energy—pronounced "chee") and making sure it is symmetrical as it flows through your body. Once your qi is increased and symmetrical, specific problems should resolve over time.

- **Meditation:** Meditation is among the most useful approaches to pain treatment. It's easy to learn, completely safe with no side effects, easy to practice, and it prevents chronic pain from promoting harmful neuroplasticity such as complex regional pain syndrome (CRPS; see page 83). Meditation quiets the mind by focusing your thoughts intently on a word, thought, object, or movement. The more you practice meditation, the better you become.

- **Self-hypnosis:** A lot of people think they cannot be hypnotized, let alone self-hypnotized, but the truth is that almost everyone can. The power of hypnosis is that you use suggestions that isolate the pain in a way that reduces its intensity. Similar to meditation, it is easy to learn and can be used throughout your life.

- **Biofeedback:** Biofeedback involves providing a person with physiologic information while performing a movement or functional task. It's useful to learn to control what is usually an involuntary process. It can be used to prevent simultaneous activation of two muscles that normally oppose each other when making a movement. For example, my injury caused me to contract both my biceps and triceps muscles when I tried to bring a fork to my mouth, when only the biceps should be active. I learned how to stop using the triceps by observing the activity of the muscles with electrodes that generated lines of force on a screen, in a technique called electromyographic (EMG) feedback. This decreased the work of my biceps so that it was less likely to be painful due to overuse.

- **Yoga:** Through its three main components (postures, breathing, and meditation), yoga can improve your physical health (fitness, balance, flexibility, and strength), mental health (by reducing stress and anxiety), and overall quality of life. The ability to achieve the postures is less important than the focus it requires to perform them—even if your attempt doesn't look pretty!

- **Massage:** Massage decreases pain both directly and indirectly. While there are different approaches to therapeutic massage, the basics include muscle compression and stroking. Compression stimulates circulation, which helps promote muscle relaxation. Stroking (long slow movements along the muscles) enhances relaxation. For me, massage has the best effect on my back, since my spinal erectors (the muscles that hold you upright and rotate the back) become tight from my sitting all day in a wheelchair.

Devices

Transcutaneous electrical nerve stimulation (TENS) uses brief electrical pulses to stimulate nerve excitation which, over time, diminishes the transmission of pain.[12] A typical battery-operated TENS unit (Figure 12) is connected to the skin using four electrodes.

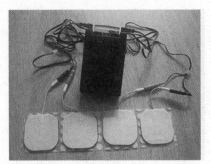

Figure 12. TENS unit

The unit can deliver electrical signals of different pulse width, frequency and intensity. For pain, TENS is usually set to a high frequency (>50 Hz = 50 times per minute) with an intensity below muscle contraction. The location of the electrodes can also be adjusted to achieve maximal pain relief.

Invasive Therapies

The three most common invasive approaches are injections of lidocaine to induce nerve block, spinal cord electrical stimulation (SCS), and intrathecal drug delivery (IDD), also known as the "pain pump."[13] Local injection of lidocaine and corticosteroids to decrease inflammation is effective for short-term pain relief only. SCS and IDD are longer-term approaches with high success rates. SCS is based on the concept that stimulating touch or vibration nerves can decrease input from pain nerves. The SCS device consists of several parts (Figure 13A): stimulating electrodes implanted in the epidural space of the spinal cord, wires that connect the electrodes to a generator, an electrical signal generator implanted in the lower abdominal area, and a remote control that you use to alter the intensity of stimulation. An X-ray of an SCS device is shown in Figure 13B. Each black rectangle is a small electrode placed under the vertebrae that represent the dermatomes from which pain arises. SCS is effective in at least 50 percent of patients, measured by a two-point reduction in pain on the ten-point scale and a decrease in pain medication dosage.

A newer technology is dorsal root ganglia (DRG) stimulation. The DRG are collections of sensory nerve cell bodies within the epidural space. In the DRG, sensory signals from a specific area of the body communicate with the nerve roots to enable spatial location of pain. Therefore, stimulation of the DRG provides therapy to a specific area that may be difficult to treat with SCS, including the hand, chest, abdomen, foot, knee, or groin. It is also

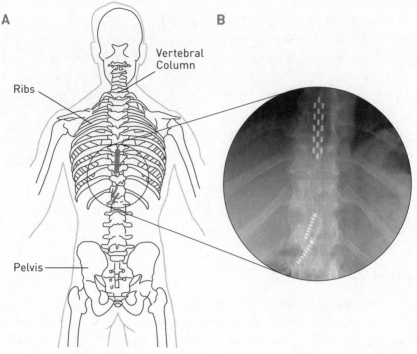

A   B

Vertebral
Column

Ribs

Pelvis

Figure 13: Spinal cord stimulation

easier to program, fewer patients have discomfort due to paresthesia, and there is less variation due to position. Future advances in technology (see chapter 19) are likely to make this approach more effective.

For IDD, a pump steadily infuses drugs into the space surrounding the spinal cord, which then flow up to the brain through the cerebrospinal fluid. There is a 70 to 90 percent success rate among patients who undergo this procedure, usually because higher doses of pain medications can be given without systemic effects.[14] At present, the FDA has approved morphine, baclofen, and ziconotide for IDD.

Common Pain Syndromes and Treatments

Central Pain Syndrome. Central pain syndrome may be the most problematic type of pain experienced after injury.[15] It's caused by damage to the nervous system, which causes increased sensitivity to pain generated in the brain (rather than the spinal cord or peripheral nerves). After stroke or TBI, it most frequently occurs in the face, and after SCI it may occur anywhere, although it most commonly appears at the level of the injury. Central pain can be constant or periodic. It is frequently described as pins and needles, shooting or jabbing, or burning. Symptoms include increased pain (sometimes, even a non-painful stimulus, such as bending my arm, will cause me pain). Treatment may be difficult, because drugs must cross the blood-brain barrier and the specific receptor pathways remain unknown. The three classes of drugs used are carbamazepine (for seizures), nortriptyline (for depression), and gabapentin (for neuropathic pain).

Complex Regional Pain Syndrome (CRPS). CRPS is a chronic systemic disease characterized by pain, edema (swelling), and changes in skin appearance.[16] The cause is unknown but likely involves inflammation, nerve damage, abnormalities in the autonomic nervous system, and increased activity of the central nervous system. Because ANI patients have these exact problems, episodes of CRPS occur in more than half of them; and many will develop it more than once. I've had it three times over seven years in my right arm, the limb most significantly impaired by my injury. To improve CRPS and achieve long-lasting results, you'll need to take a multidisciplinary approach, starting by meeting with your physiatrist. Pain reduction is the first priority. Your doctor will be able to present you with a wide variety of therapies and suggest how to use them in combination for the best effects. For example, heat treatment and transcutaneous electrical nerve stimulation (TENS) are both effective at pain management, and may be helpful for you. Edema is best treated with a combination of elevation, massage (especially lymphatic drainage), and compression. Your doctor will also likely recommend cardiovascular exercise—which, for me, is the most effective treatment.

Your routine should include both active range of motion (ROM) exercises within the pain-free range to regain function, along with stress loading and traction. Stress loading involves applying weight to the affected limb frequently during the day. I usually lean on my right forearm on top of my wheelchair's arm for five to ten minutes every hour. Traction requires a weight and a pulley. The simplest setup is to have the pulley hanging on the top of a closed door, with a ring for you to hold on one side of the pulley and a weight on the other side. Holding on to the ring for five to ten minutes three or four times daily strengthens the bones and muscles in your arm. Over time, you increase the weight as you improve. I find this traction exercise less useful than other exercises, because most devices use a water-filled bag as the weight (I worry about leaking), finding the right door is not easy (it needs clearance on top), and it can be uncomfortable. Mirror box therapy (see Figure 8; page 47) can be a useful addition to exercise therapy in addressing CRPS. Several drugs can be used to treat CRPS, including antidepressants; anti-inflammatories, such as corticosteroids and NSAIDs; gabapentin and pregabalin; and opioids. The goal should be short-term use. I've found corticosteroids to be most effective, starting with 60 mg/day and a slow tapering off over two weeks.

Keep Going!

Reducing your pain in ways that allow you to enjoy time with family and friends and help you participate in physical, occupational, speech, and other therapies is an essential goal, not a luxury. Furthermore, if you are experiencing pain frequently, you may associate this pain with rehabilitation and thereby reduce your willingness to perform physical and occupational therapy. Make sure this subject is one you and your family raise with your health care team as soon as possible; your mental and physical recovery depend on it.

Everything You Need to Know

Pain is one of the most common consequences of ANI. Unaddressed, it damages your quality of life, and limits your ability to achieve your recovery and rehabilitation goals.

Successful pain management requires a multidisciplinary approach, active monitoring and adjustment of your pain medications, and a willingness to try pain relief techniques besides drugs, such as cognitive behavioral therapy, meditation, exercise, self-hypnosis, and more.

Early on, consult with a physiatrist or pain specialist who has expertise in regaining function while managing pain.

Your goal in pain management should be to find yourself relying less on drugs and more on other therapies as you recover physical strength, range of motion, and mental resilience.

Keep a journal of everything you do to address your pain, and keep the conversation going with your care team. Achieving successful pain management is an ongoing process.

Rehabilitation: Slow and Steady Wins the Race

*Five Steps to Getting the Most from
Rehabilitation and Restoration Therapies*

M Y FIRST GOAL IN rehabilitation was to improve my independence. I wanted to be able to do the "big" things, like getting in and out of bed, or on and off the toilet, on my own—and *ASAP*. But this goal changed as I took a more careful look at my day-to-day needs. Meals were essential, and I couldn't feed myself. As I envisioned my life at home, I didn't like imagining my wife spoon-feeding me, and knew it would add one more burden— three times a day, seven days a week—to her already overloaded schedule. As eager as I was to regain some of my dignity in the bathroom, I decided that being able to feed myself independently would be my number one priority.

My injury had made it difficult for me to swallow, because some of the muscles and nerves that coordinate swallowing were not working after my injury. Even after my ventilator was removed, I wasn't allowed to eat, because I was at risk for aspiration pneumonia. This is a serious complication in which food, during swallowing (the food bolus in blue), partially goes down the trachea under the epiglottis—not down the esophagus like nor-

mal (Figure 14). Dys- phagia (difficulty swal- lowing) is a common problem, so it's possible that your rehab will include relearning how to swallow.

Thanks to my ther- apy team, my ability to swallow eventually improved enough for

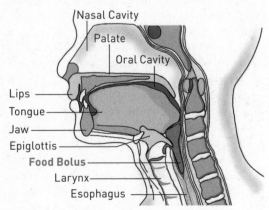

Figure 14: Aspiration pneumonia

me to eat solid food. With that accomplishment behind me and the limited use I had gained in one arm, I was in a rush to start using utensils, especially a fork and a knife. But I was too weak (and clumsy) to hold a fork and bring food to my mouth. It was frustrating to spend several *minutes* trying to stab a single piece of food—only to have it fall off my fork. More food landed in my lap than made it into my mouth, so after every meal I would need to change my clothes. After two weeks of trying, I decided to hold off on eating independently until I was physically strong enough, which turned out to take almost three months.

This chapter is all about helping you get the most out of the physical, occupational, speech, psychiatric, and other therapies that are part of getting back to life after injury. The goal of rehabilitation specialists is to find ways to *improve your quality of life*. By working with your existing capabilities and deficits, your therapy team will help you develop your functional abilities to their fullest extent, and teach you adaptive behaviors as well. There's no set timetable or formula for rehabilitation, but the objective is always the same: to help you achieve the ability to enjoy a full life as independently as possible.

Aphasia and Balance

If you have suffered a stroke or TBI and have been left with aphasia (difficulty with verbal and written communication), improving your ability to speak and to understand others is likely your number one goal. The frustration of not being able to communicate your needs or, even worse, not being able to understand what people are saying, is significant and can lead to a devastating sense of isolation. Your neurologist should be someone who has expertise in aphasia, and they will refer you to a speech therapist (also called a speech pathologist) who specializes in aphasia. If you live in or near a city, these providers will be able to recommend an aphasia group for you to attend (be sure to ask about it if your providers don't mention it). These gatherings, which are led by an experienced speech therapist with a specialty in aphasia, are an excellent way to enhance your rehabilitation. Your fellow participants will also be experiencing aphasia and will be at different stages of recovery. In this supportive environment, you will make progress toward your goal while benefiting from the inspiration and experiences of others in the group.

If you have experienced a TBI, your top priority might be improving your balance. Among other things, TBI can result in sensory loss and dizziness. These changes predispose you to falls and injuries, so working on improved balance and visual cues may be the most important initial goal for you.

Your Rehabilitation Program: The Five-Step Plan

As you embark on your rehabilitation, the following five steps will help set the stage for success. You will: 1) determine your personal goals; 2) prepare yourself mentally; 3) make a schedule; 4) practice, practice, practice; and 5) establish how to pay for your rehabilitative services. Let's look at each one.

1. **Identify your goals (and what stands in the way of reaching them).** All ANIs affect multiple organ systems, because the brain and spinal cord control the function of all organ systems. Therefore, rehab must be multidisciplinary and it requires a team to provide appropriate care. For example, I performed OT and PT every day, with special sessions on shoulder therapy. I also saw a speech-language pathologist (SLP) three times a week to help me with swallowing. I was fortunate that my speech, vision, and language processing were not affected by my injury. These can be the major problems in people with stroke and TBI. When setting out on your rehabilitation journey, consider which functions are the most important for you to regain. Start by writing a list of your goals in a dedicated rehab book or spreadsheet, and then prioritize them by asking yourself this question: *Which ones would make the greatest difference to my quality of life?* The one that lands at the top is where you should begin. Discuss that goal with your therapy team—they can help you figure out which goals are most achievable, and in what order. Remember that success generates more success, so make your first goal attainable. Keep in mind, though, that your priorities can change along the way, as mine did. That's OK; it's all part of the journey.

2. **Prepare yourself mentally (believe in and *visualize* your success).** As we saw in chapter 2, the connection between the body and the mind is astoundingly powerful. Professional athletes have long worked with sports psychologists and used visualization to mentally rehearse their performances. This successful technique can also be useful in your rehabilitation. Visualization involves creating a mental image of what you want to see yourself doing and/or feeling. And repetition is important. When you "watch" the images in your mind over and over, you are actually training your mind and body to be more successful at the task. That's why you must *visualize* success. The ability to imagine achieving a difficult physical task is fundamental

to successful rehabilitation. There are three essential tactics: mental rehearsal of the task, relaxation, and emotional control.

- **Mental rehearsal is imagining yourself performing the task as carefully as you can.** I watched YouTube videos of people learning to walk again, which made it easier to visualize doing this myself. In the future, virtual reality goggles will make it so you'll be able to see yourself walking in a much more realistic manner, which will be much better for visualizing.

- **Mental relaxation is an important component of visualizing your achievement of a goal.** Great athletes compete in a state of relaxation, and the same idea applies to your rehabilitation. Eliud Kipchoge, a Kenyan long-distance runner, is the first person ever to run a marathon in under two hours. When asked how he did it, he said, "I was really calm. . . . I have been training for this for four and a half months. I have been putting my heart and mind to run under two hours for a marathon."[1] His approach to a huge physical challenge was to train his mind and his body to be relaxed. You can achieve this state with the same techniques: practicing visualization in a relaxed state and focusing your thoughts on reaching the goal.

- **Emotional control is primarily about decreasing your fear through conditioning and practice.** When I was learning to walk again, taking the first step using my platform walker made me extremely anxious, because I was afraid of falling. My therapist helped by holding and steadying me as I took one step forward. I repeated this many times until I was comfortable enough to maintain almost all my weight on one foot. Walking can also be practiced with a robot that assists your legs and holds you up, a treadmill with body support and therapists moving your legs, or an overhead body weight support system that prevents you from falling.

Remember that your therapists can best assist you because they know your abilities better than anyone. They know your strength, balance, and the range of movements that you can attempt safely. Their guidance is invaluable, because if you hurt yourself, you will set yourself back weeks or even months. That's why slow and steady always wins the race.

3. **Set a schedule and stick to it (and put it in writing).** No matter how hectic your life may be, set a schedule for your rehabilitation therapies and stick to it. Each type of therapy will be targeted at specific goals; be sure to record each of your sessions and keep track of your progress. Whether you are the person writing down the schedule and goals or they are being written and updated by someone else in your household, having a written log is valuable. Describing your goals in *written* form is strongly associated with success in attaining them; in fact, putting pen to paper makes it more than four times as likely that you will reach your objectives.[2] When you write things down, you have something tangible to look at as a reminder—every day, if you make looking at the calendar/notebook a daily event. Neuropsychologists say this visual cue influences your determination to get something done. When you keep a notebook, you are creating a picture in your mind, which makes your mind more efficient when it focuses on the important stuff.

4. **Practice makes perfect.** It will require thousands of repetitions for you to master some of the skills and goals on your list. In other words, becoming good at something requires practice—and lots of it. When you are working to recover from your injury, you will need to relearn things you used to do without thinking, by practicing the exercises your therapists teach you, again and again.

   What's going to motivate you to practice so intensively? For me, it was my strong desire to be a participant in family holiday traditions throughout the year. Those gatherings are filled with happiness, joy, love, and laughter. So it was wonderfully helpful when my daughter taped large photos of my grandchildren to the wall facing my bed. Looking at those smiling, hopeful faces every morning gave me the strength to keep going, no matter how discouraged I was or how much pain I was in. Identify a big motivator (or two) of your own and use that as you become dedicated to a heavy-duty routine of practice, practice, and more practice.

   Insurance companies and most doctors recommend that rehabilitation should be continued until you reach a plateau, which varies greatly among people. Rehabilitation is tightly linked to neurological recovery, which depends significantly on the severity of your injury. In general, most patients have their most rapid recovery early on (one to three months), with a slowing in recovery over time. But I firmly believe that you can still recover significantly over time, by continuously performing general strengthening and range of motion exercises as well as specific tasks. For example, I stretch and lift weights, primarily for my upper body, three times a week and practice holding a wine glass, using eating utensils, brushing my teeth, and opening the mail (with a letter opener).

5. **Determine where to perform rehab after discharge and how to pay for it.** The facility for rehabilitation after discharge should be based on your degree of independence in activities of daily living (ADL). If you have mild functional impairment, you will likely do well at home with home health care or outpatient follow-up. For example, when I left Kessler, I wasn't ready to go home, because I had not developed a reliable bowel program and could not transfer from my bed without a Hoyer lift (Figure 37; see page 216). If I had been more independent, I could have gone to a skilled nursing facility. Instead, I remained a patient in a rehab unit of Strong Memorial Hospital. This enabled me to continue three hours of OT and PT each day while I worked with an aide who would later join me at home every morning and night to assist me with personal care and eating. It took me nineteen days to master the tasks necessary for me to live comfortably and safely at home.

The doctor overseeing your care in the hospital will refer you to the outpatient services you will need after discharge and the therapists who will work with you as part of your rehabilitation. As discussed in chapter 3, you'll need referrals and a prescription for specific rehab therapies, if you want your insurance plan to pay for your care. Keep a notebook where you write down every interaction with your insurer. Your choice of insurer will be largely determined by your employment status and financial resources. The most likely ones will be your employer's insurance plan, public insurance (Medicaid, Medicare, and SSDI), disability insurance, your local for-profit (e.g., Aetna, and United Health Group) and not-for-profit health insurers (e.g., Blue Cross/Blue Shield, and Kaiser Permanente), and life insurance.

The Social Security Administration (SSA) offers disability benefits, including those for military veterans whose disability resulted from service injuries. The SSA also offers information on how to make the most of your benefits if you choose to continue working, so you can use this compensation to pay for necessities like home modifications. If you are sixty or older, your local senior center will likely have an expert on SSA who meets (for free) with anyone who needs help getting information. You can also attend free presentations on Social Security benefits at your local public library.

Explore free community resources that can help you and your family if there are gaps in your insurance policy. If you live near a university or medical school, you may be able to take advantage of the hands-on clinical hours that students in rehabilitation therapy programs are required to complete (including occupational, physical, and speech therapy). You may also be able to use the school's fitness center at no charge—something we offer at the University of Rochester Medical Center—where exercise physiologists will help you plan a workout routine.

There are foundations across the country that support people with disabilities, with chapters in many communities. Usually, their focus is on supplying durable medical equipment needs such as wheelchairs, hospital beds, shower chairs, standing frames, electronic devices, and so on (see chapter 15 for more on this). Some nonprofit organizations are committed to providing money to help pay for the cost of renovating a home bathroom to be accessible, for example, or installing an exterior ramp for a wheelchair. Others have funds designated for things like specialized wheelchairs for sports, hand bicycles, or sit-skis for snow and water skiing. You'll find a list of these organizations in the Resources section at the back of this book.

There are several ways to reduce the costs of your recovery and rehabilitation. To keep the cost of drugs down, you can buy generic drugs whenever possible and use mail-order pharmacies for a three-month supply at a time. If you qualify for public insurance, these programs offer rehabilitation for free or with a small copayment. If you are a veteran, medications, doctors' visits, rehabilitation therapy, and durable medical equipment are free at your local VA hospital. And if you're fortunate to live near a school that has rehabilitation programs, you can have access at no cost to students who are learning clinical skills. Finally, you can volunteer for clinical trials, many of which have a rehabilitation component, at no cost.

It's also a good idea to understand the *purpose* of each drug prescribed for you. Talk to your physiatrist and your primary care physician about which drugs you can reduce or eliminate. After living with my injury for more than ten years, I've managed to switch to generic drugs almost exclusively and have eliminated many others. The savings have been significant.

Continuous Rehabilitation Can Lead to Regaining More Functional Abilities

Rehabilitation is a long-term goal. I schedule and devote a significant amount of time to rehab activities each week—even all these years after my injury—and I continue to improve my functional abilities because of it. I may be unusual in the extent of my recovery, but I believe that everyone can regain function by working continuously on their rehabilitation.

I believe that my determination and organization have helped me get to where I am today. But I also have my down days, when I am so painfully aware of my limitations. I've emerged enough times from these significant disability periods to know that there is light at the end of the tunnel. So, it's important to stay resilient. I don't expect you to follow my schedule; I just want you to set your own goals, schedule therapy, and stick to it. Once you commit to a schedule, you are on your way to a better quality of life. Yes, it's going to take time and effort, but regaining function is worth it.

True Grit

Rehabilitation is hard. There's no way to sugarcoat it. And there's no way to avoid it either. A quote attributed to Winston Churchill states, "When you're going through hell, keep going." That thought epitomizes my approach to rehab. Yes, some of it is hell. But I know from experience that with grit, determination, and resilience, you'll keep going, too.

Resilience comes from within. When you overcome challenges and learn that you can change yourself and your environment to solve problems, you've tapped into your innate resilience. It's more than confidence; it's conquering your fear and self-doubt. When you face these difficult moments, reach down deep and use the power of your mind, and you will prevail.

Of course, your journey will be aided by the people around you, friends and family who believe in you. Don't be reluctant to accept their love and support. It's a lifeline for you and deeply gratifying for them. One of my best sources of uplifting encouragement is a group of four paraplegics; these buddies of mine have all been in wheelchairs for more than twenty-five years—more than twice as long as I have. We call ourselves the Push Men, and we meet for dinner every few months. Each person's wisdom and understanding, gained by many years of dealing with disability, makes us a powerful source of support and inspiration for each other.

I believe in you. I hope this book empowers you to do the same. And, now that you're equipped to make the most of your rehabilitation, you can begin to focus on living your healthiest lifestyle.

————

Everything You Need to Know

Approach rehabilitation with optimism and the knowledge that progress may be slower than expected. Use the following five steps to help you as you work to get your brain and body back:

- Determine your personal goals.
- Prepare yourself mentally.
- Make a schedule and put it in writing.
- Practice, practice, and practice.
- Establish how to pay for your rehabilitative services.

Along the way, be open to accepting all the help, love, and support offered to you.

Your Lifestyle = Your State of Wellness

How to Strengthen Good Habits and Lose the Ones that Zap Your Health

I'VE BEEN A FITNESS ENTHUSIAST my whole life. Before my accident, my idea of Saturday morning fun was a sixty-mile bike ride. I worked out with weights, skied, and followed a healthy Mediterranean diet. Taking care of my body was an integral part of my routine, and it made me feel good, too. After I suffered my injury, however, I knew that all of my favorite strenuous activities would be a thing of the past. I also knew that a healthy lifestyle would be more important than ever for my longevity—and for any chance I had at getting my brain and body back.

Your lifestyle—what you choose to eat and drink, how much sleep you get, how physically active you are, how much alcohol you consume, whether or not you are a smoker, and how you react to stress—is the foundation of your overall state of health. Lifestyle is a huge factor in lifespan and in your quality of life, too. And post-injury, these factors can enhance or hinder your recovery. So now is the time to make adjustments that will strengthen your good habits and free you of the ones that may be eroding your health.

You Are What You Eat

A healthy diet is an important source of nutrition and the best way to maintain an optimal weight. What is a healthy diet? Generally speaking, it includes fruits and vegetables, healthy fats, protein, and plenty of fiber, which can be found in whole grains and legumes. There are lots of "healthy" diets being promoted every year—so many, actually, that it can be confusing as to what you *should* eat. But there are good ones that stand the test of time. The two I always recommend are the DASH diet and the Mediterranean diet.

The DASH diet (Dietary Approaches to Stop Hypertension) is recommended by the American Heart Association and the National Institutes of Health.[1] It was designed to prevent hypertension by limiting sodium intake (less than 2,300 mg per day). Because hypertension is common in SCI survivors and present in more than 50 percent of stroke survivors, the DASH diet is applicable to many people with ANI.

The Mediterranean diet is based on the traditional foods of the regions along the Mediterranean Sea, particularly the island of Sicily.[2] Studies have found that these populations have a very low incidence of obesity and chronic disease (such as type 2 diabetes, heart disease, cancer, and lung disease) and have excellent longevity. Both of these diets call for foods that are easy to find, decrease the risk of heart attack and stroke, and include options to suit a variety of tastes and budgets. Recommendations include at least five servings of fruits and vegetables a day; at least 25 grams of fiber; whole grains rather than highly processed ones; low-fat dairy products; legumes, poultry, and seafood for protein; and limited consumption of red meat.

There are many books that present diets for optimal health in recovery. These include Dr. Michael Greger's *How Not to Die*, which focuses on preventing and treating the top fifteen causes of death in the US; Dr. Jason Fung's *The Obesity Code*, which discusses a five-step approach to diet that focuses on hormones, appetite, insulin resistance, and fat storage; and Dorothy Calimeris's *The Complete Anti-Inflammatory Diet for Beginners*, which discusses the harmful effects of foods that increase inflammation versus foods that are beneficial for treating inflammation (fruits and vegetables, whole grains, plant-based proteins, fish, and fresh herbs and spices). You can find more about these diets and recipes in books or online (see Resources on page 282).

Consult with a Nutritionist

Even if you are at an ideal weight, ask for a consultation with a registered nutritionist at the hospital. They will assess your eating habits and help you design a diet that will continue to support your health, even if your ability to eat has changed. After an ANI, it's particularly important to achieve and maintain your ideal weight, especially if your mobility has been adversely affected, since excess weight will make your rehabilitation more difficult. Being overweight also puts you at greater risk for serious health problems, including type 2 diabetes, heart disease, and cancer.

If you are employed at a large company, you may benefit from an employee health program, which usually includes free consultation with a nutritionist. Your primary care physician can also refer you to a local community wellness program that includes dietary counseling, which may be covered by your health insurance or may even be free.

Alcohol and ANI

Your consumption of alcohol may need to change after your injury. After TBI, significant research data shows that you should not consume any alcohol for at least one year, due to decreased functional recovery. While similar data does not exist for stroke and SCI, you may find that limiting your alcohol consumption is best for your health and recovery.

If you regularly exceeded the recommended daily amount of alcohol (one drink per day for women, and two for men) pre-injury, you may need help cutting back or eliminating alcohol. Let your doctor know if you want help. Your doctor and nutritionist can counsel you on how much alcohol you should be drinking, if any. They can also refer you to a program to help you stop drinking if it's a problem for you to do so on your own. See page 33 for more.

Supplements

The standards for the amounts and types of food, minerals, and vitamins that should be consumed daily by Americans are established by the National Academy of Sciences, National Research Council, and the National Academy of Medicine. Most doctors and dieticians use the Recommended Daily Allowance (RDA)—which is the average daily intake sufficient to meet the dietary requirement of nearly all healthy people—when considering the best eating plan for ANI patients. RDA is listed by age, sex, and activity level in *A Consumer's Guide to the DRIs (Dietary Reference Intakes)*, as published by Health Canada.[3]

A healthy diet alone should meet the RDA standards, which is why I don't generally recommend supplements. But vitamin D is one notable exception. Low levels of vitamin D can contribute to osteoporosis and consequently an increased risk of fractures. Since you may be more susceptible to falls and, therefore, fractures, I recommend that you ask to be tested for 25-hydroxyvitamin D_3 levels while you are in the hospital. If your levels are low, start daily supplementation with at least 1,000 units of vitamin D_3. Your doctor should schedule follow-up lab work to monitor the effects of the supplements.

If you are meeting RDA standards through diet, you will likely not need to take herbal supplements either. These supplements, which include coenzyme Q10, echinacea, and melatonin (more on this in chapter 8), can be problematic due to inaccurate labeling, and the presence of other active compounds that are not identified on the label. If you decide to start or continue herbal supplements, be sure to inform your doctor, as they can interfere with some prescription drugs.

Physical Activity

After your injury, it's especially important to get regular physical exercise, to the extent that you can, as you recover. Work with your therapy team to develop an exercise program that increases your flexibility, balance, and strength—these are the key components to ongoing rehabilitation.

Your exercise routine should include both aerobic and strength-building activities. As you recover, regular exercise will help you increase your mobility and independence, enhance your mood, and improve your mental health. Physical fitness is also beneficial for disease prevention. It reduces your risk of cardiovascular disease, heart attack, stroke, type 2 diabetes, and more. Even modest amounts of regular physical activity, such as walking or using a hand cycle for thirty minutes every day, deliver a significant benefit.

When you are discharged from outpatient physical therapy, be sure to ask your therapist to write down the exercises and competitive sports in which you can participate. There are formal guidelines for TBI patients with concussions on returning to school and to sports, available on the websites of the Centers for Disease Control and Prevention (CDC) and the Brain Injury Association of America (BIAA).[4] For stroke survivors, it's important not to overexercise, because the parts of the brain that are still recovering may not get enough oxygen. While you can continue to work out at home, you may also want to schedule time with a personal trainer at a local fitness center, which may be covered by your health insurance policy. The trainer can help you stay on track with your fitness goals and tweak your routine to challenge your body. If you live near a university, you may be able to take advantage of a free training plan developed by an exercise physiologist just for you. Ask your physical therapist about this before you are discharged.

No matter where you live, you can make physical activity part of your day. There are fitness apps that you can download for free or for a small fee, and there are some excellent workout videos (also free) on YouTube. You'll find a list in the Resources on page 284.

Your Ideal Weight

Ensuring that you are at your ideal weight will improve your health and recovery. Being overweight puts you at increased risk of cancer, heart disease, diabetes, and orthopedic problems. If you are not yet at that optimal weight, weight loss is best achieved using multiple approaches, including behavioral therapy, diet, and physical activity. Maintaining an ideal weight will make it easier for you to transfer in and out of a wheelchair, which will decrease the likelihood of pressure ulcers (see chapter 13). It will also make it easier to get around if you are using a cane, walker, or wheelchair. In particular, our shoulders were not designed to bear heavy loads, which occurs with any of these assistive devices, so many people will develop significant shoulder problems, especially with the rotator cuff, as they age. Maintaining your ideal weight also means you can purchase equipment that is less expensive, since extra weight requires larger adaptive devices with more strength.

Smoking

Everyone knows that smoking is harmful to health. It's linked to cancer, lung disease, and heart disease. And after an ANI, smoking is even more dangerous. Smoking damages lung function, and if you've had a traumatic brain injury or spinal cord injury at C5 or above, your diaphragm function is impaired, putting you at increased risk for pneumonia.

Smoking decreases bone mass and increases the risk of hip fracture, especially in women. If you do not perform regular weight-bearing activities, such as walking, you can develop osteoporosis and subsequently will be at much greater risk of bone fractures from even a simple fall.

Quitting can be difficult, but there are successful programs out there, most of them covered by health insurance. (Even if you have to pay out of pocket, think of what you spend each week on cigarettes and how much you'll save once you quit!) Some programs combine behavioral therapy with prescription drugs or over-the-counter products that reduce cravings for nicotine. Hypnosis has proven to be a highly successful tactic, even for long-term smokers. There are also free telephone quit lines (like 1-800-QUIT-NOW), text messaging programs, and apps. Talk to your health care provider about your options.

You can get started by not allowing any smoking in your house. Pick a date to quit smoking, put it on the calendar, and tell your loved ones about your plan. Quitting smoking will take effort, but it's well worth it. And even if you fail to stay smoke-free after your first try, the likelihood of being successful increases every time you try to quit. So, keep trying!

Stress

It's impossible to lead a stress-free life. And when it comes to stressful experiences, ANI is off-the-charts. That's exactly why it's important to learn coping strategies and skills that will lessen the impact stress has on your day-to-day life. There are three therapies I recommend for chronic stress and anxiety: 1) cognitive behavioral therapy (CBT), which, as we learned in chapter 2, includes techniques such as relaxation training, identification of stressful situations, and using images to decrease stress response; 2) mind/body therapies, such as yoga, tai chi, meditation, and mindfulness (which you will learn about in chapter 8), which can reduce anxiety and depression; and 3) exercise and increased physical activity (my preferred approach!). These therapies will be lifelong tools you can use to improve your health, your relationships with loved ones, and your quality of life.

Try to avoid treating your stress with drugs as much as possible. Relying on drugs can mean that you end up in a vicious cycle of taking the drug to relax, discontinuing the drug because you feel better, and then experiencing a rebound of stress, forcing you to restart the drug. That said, if you remain anxious and stressed even with exercise, mind-body therapies, and CBT, regular low-dose prophylactic treatment with SSRIs or SNRIs can be useful (see chapter 4). Avoid benzodiazepines, like Valium, because they frequently cause mild cognitive impairment.

Sleep

Sleep is when the body rests, repairs, and restores itself. Adults need seven to eight hours of quality sleep (uninterrupted sleep in a quiet, dark, comfortable environment) per night. Good sleep habits protect your cardiac health, your blood pressure, and even your weight. A lack of sufficient sleep can exacerbate existing type 2 diabetes and can even initiate it (the same is true for high blood pressure); it can also alter the balance of the two important weight-regulating hormones—leptin and ghrelin—leading to weight gain.

After ANI, it's crucial to establish a quality sleep routine. Sleep disturbances can be common, especially if your injury damaged parts of the brain that are important for sleep. Chronic pain, mental health disorders (especially anxiety and PTSD), and neuropathic sensations such as numbness, electric shocks, and skin sensitivity—all common aftereffects of ANI—can also worsen sleep. In addition, many medications can cause daytime drowsiness and frequent napping, making it difficult to sleep for seven or eight consecutive hours at night.

After ANI (especially stroke and TBI), sleep disorders—including insomnia, obstructive sleep apnea, and central sleep apnea—are very common, affecting more than 60 percent of people.[5] Sleep apnea is characterized by pauses in breathing or periods of extremely shallow breathing during sleep, decreasing the amount of oxygen in your blood. Untreated, sleep apnea increases the risk of heart attack, stroke, type 2 diabetes, heart failure, irregular heartbeat, obesity, erectile dysfunction, and serious car accidents (every year, untreated sleep apnea is responsible for thousands of drivers falling asleep at the wheel). Sleep apnea is usually treated with continuous positive airway pressure (CPAP) that maintains the open airways from your from your nose, mouth, and pharynx. It is highly effective, but many people have difficulty sleeping with a mask and the noise of a CPAP machine.[6] Psychotherapy-based approaches are also effective for treating sleep disturbances after TBI.[7] Acupuncture has been shown to improve insomnia following stroke, and sleep disturbances after TBI.[8]

Be sure to talk with your doctor about the quality of your sleep, including how many hours per night you sleep, if you snore loudly every night, and if you find yourself dozing off unintentionally during the day. Your doctor will then be able to diagnose sleep apnea from an overnight sleep study at home or in an accredited sleep lab. This sleep study should be covered by insurance, as is treatment, and your pulmonologist or sleep specialist will discuss treatment options with you. Don't put off the conversation; the contribution proper sleep makes to your quality of life and to your recovery cannot be overstated. All sleep disturbances, especially sleep apnea, contribute to fatigue, hypertension, and impaired thinking. The increase in hypertension is particularly problematic, because the risk of stroke rises in parallel with the rise in systolic blood pressure (the upper blood pressure number). Hypertension also harms the blood vessels and nerves that feed and control the bowel, bladder, and penis, as well as the process of breathing.

Achieving wellness requires daily attention to many lifestyle choices. Feeling healthy and good about yourself will enable you to be more sociable and emotionally stable. Also, as we will discuss in the next chapter, to enjoy physical intimacy.

Everything You Need to Know

Your lifestyle—the large and small choices you make on a daily basis—determines your lifelong levels of health and happiness. Use this opportunity to examine your habits and make improvements where needed. Keep at it, keep a log, enlist the help of family and friends, and be sure to take advantage of the health care professionals and community organizations that can assist you on this journey to get your brain and body back. The most important elements of your lifestyle are in the list that follows; look at each one, write your answers in your journal, and determine where you can do better:

- What do you eat and drink?
- What do you do for physical fitness?
- Are you at an ideal weight?
- Do you smoke? (It's time to quit!)
- Do you handle the stresses of life well?
- How much sleep do you get each night?

Sexual Healing

How to Address Your Sexuality,
Sexual Function, and Fertility

AFTER MY INJURY, the changes to my body image and my sense of sexuality were among the most difficult to accept. I had always taken good care of my body. I had been comfortable with my sexuality, confident in my interactions with the world and with my wife. But after my injury, the changes to my abilities as a sexual partner were emotionally and psychologically devastating. Thankfully, my rehabilitation team began addressing my sexual function on my very first day. I guess that's a pretty good indication of how important it is in the eyes of medical experts.

Physical intimacy is an essential part of life for most people. Sexual contact nourishes your mental, physical, and emotional health. Intimacy requires mutual vulnerability, which helps you grow as an individual and as a partner. The way I see it, physical intimacy is an emotional nutrient, absolutely essential to the viability of a long-lasting loving partnership. Physical intimacy is also important even if you're not in a permanent relationship; it can enhance your self-image as well as your physical and emotional well-being. I'm not alone in that perspective; according to many experts, close relationships are essential for our mental and physical health, and sexual satisfaction is key to relationship satisfaction.[1]

Sexuality: What Is It?

In my years of interacting with other people with ANIs, I've consistently found one of their earliest concerns to be the dramatic change to their sexual function. This isn't surprising, because it's a natural human desire to bond with others through physical intimacy. Your sexuality includes how you think about yourself, the desires that influence your sexual orientation, and how you express your sexuality—the way you connect emotionally with someone and how you translate that emotion into physical actions.

Sexuality also encompasses your thoughts about your body image, your sense of how attractive you are, your self-esteem, and your ease in social settings. If, after your injury, you view yourself as unattractive, unable to perform intercourse, and unable to make your partner happy, you may feel inadequate, unworthy, and burdensome to your partner. Inevitably, this creates a negative emotional state that can impair your recovery and can damage—perhaps irrevocably—your relationship. If this applies to your state of mind, please know that there are many ways to address these feelings, and knowledgeable clinicians who can help. As someone who was nearly completely paralyzed, I can assure you there *is* a way back to enjoying physical intimacy and sex.

While there may be obvious visible changes in what you see when you look in the mirror, more important is how you *feel* about your body. To become a sexual human being again after your injury, think about what you value in yourself and others. Perhaps the most critical step is to take a look at your self-esteem. It's natural to have low self-esteem when you're not able to do things for yourself. Becoming comfortable with being dependent on others and learning how to ask for help takes time, openness, and humility. Working on your self-esteem will help you to gain control over your life again and allow you to begin to feel better about who you are—including who you are sexually.

As you recover, you'll discover your physical abilities to perform in a sexual encounter. The first questions you'll need to ask are: Can I have an orgasm, and will I be able to go through the physical aspects of arousal (engorgement of the penis or clitoris) and the physical movements required for intercourse and orgasm? You can learn about your sexual ability through masturbation, assuming that your upper extremity function allows for it. You may also find creative ways to stimulate your body, even if your function is compromised. The brain is the largest sex organ; your ability to have an orgasm is determined more by what's in your head than what's in your genital area. Though an orgasm is usually associated with a physical sensation, you can experience feelings of intense pleasure without the same physical manifestations. You can develop new pathways to orgasm—by letting yourself be open to them (see page 107). And, of course, there are several drugs and devices that can facilitate the physical components of sex (see pages 112 and 114).

Physical Intimacy in a Relationship

There are ups and downs in every long-term relationship. The state of your partnership at the time of your injury is likely to carry over to your hospitalization and rehabilitation. If your relationship is already struggling, it may not be able to survive your injury. Even if your relationship is strong, it may be rocked to its core. But if you're able to achieve mutually satisfying physical intimacy, it can be one of the lifelines that pulls you—as individuals and as a couple—through this trauma.

Achieving new ways to find sexual satisfaction together will take work, honesty, a sense of humor, and a willingness to be vulnerable. It's not easy, but if you try, you may be able to strengthen your relationship and, in turn, your own recovery. I know several couples who have survived the aftermath of one partner's injury intact and now have wonderful relationships. And many people are able to find partners after their injury as well.

My Marriage and Beyond

In my own marriage, struggles with physical intimacy, sexuality, and our new roles took a toll that, ultimately, we could not overcome. After more than thirty years together, we separated and, eventually, divorced—an outcome neither one of us would have predicted. After the divorce, and with help, I was able to resolve my fears and hang-ups about my self-image, self-esteem, and sense of masculinity. As a result, I was also able to become much more positive about my *entire* rehabilitation and recovery. When things seemed too difficult, I found comfort and strength in my mantra: *Forgive, let it go, and move on.*

Dating: How do I get people to look past the wheelchair?

The process of dating can be hard work and may not be much fun. This is especially true if you use a wheelchair, because all of the usual dating routines—going out to dinner, attending concerts or plays, and even visiting your partner's home—will be changed, especially if these places aren't wheelchair-accessible. Even if you're not in a wheelchair, the changes in your behavior, self-esteem, and your physical limitations may make your dating life unusual. For example, I have a good friend who needs someone to drive him around. With some regularity, the driver participates in the conversations between him and his date, which can make things awkward.

Dating After an ANI

When I decided to start dating again after my divorce, I asked my married friends to invite a single friend of theirs to join us all for dinner. My hope was that the familiarity of being among friends would lessen the tension of a first date. It did. But it was a painfully slow strategy, because my friends didn't like being my matchmaker. Even worse, they really didn't know what kind of person I was looking for—probably because I had no idea myself. After being in one relationship for thirty years, I had no idea how to date, especially not with my new physical limitations. After three such "dates," I realized I was doomed to another ninety-seven bad experiences (I had promised myself that I would go on a maximum of one hundred dates).

The two other options I had were to ask someone out on a date myself or to try an online dating service. I had accumulated a few names since my divorce, so I called one of them—Dr. Coral Surgeon—to see if she was willing to go on a date, and she said yes. We agreed to double-date with a couple with whom we were both very friendly, but unfortunately, that date never happened, because the other couple had a family emergency. Though we were both nervous to get together alone, we ultimately decided that we had nothing to lose. When we went to dinner, we discovered that we had much in common—to start, we both liked red wine, fish, and rum raisin ice cream. We also found, over time, that we shared similar values, such as love of family, hard work, caring for those in need, participating actively in our community, and a love of the arts (especially dance and painting). Most important, we could talk about any topic, however personal or difficult, with relative ease. This ability to communicate openly, and not avoid issues has paved the way to a successful marriage and has enabled us to enjoy a vibrant and loving relationship for the past eight years.

In speaking with friends since then, I've learned that online dating is often a much better option for most people. It will certainly give you a much larger number of people to choose from. There are "general" dating apps and websites, and there are specialized websites for people with particular interests. Several focus on people in wheelchairs and other disabilities. Make sure that your profile mentions that you are disabled and use a wheelchair or a walker; being honest will start the date in the right direction.

Before venturing into the dating world, it may help to reevaluate. Looking good and feeling good about yourself are certainly good places to start. Develop your own style, one that fits your new status in a wheelchair (if you use one), by purchasing new, wheelchair-appropriate attire or altering your existing clothes (more on this on page 214). For example, I stopped wearing regular overcoats and had a tailor modify my overcoats to become capes. At one point, I thought, *Just add a cap and you could look like Sherlock Holmes!* If you believe in who you are, it's easy to be attractive to others. And being outgoing and friendly will help you find success dating. Be the person who starts conversations. Get out and do activities that bring you in contact with people who share your interests.

Can We Talk?

One of the most important components of satisfying physical intimacy is the ability of both partners to engage in open, honest discussions about it. After your injury, that ability becomes even more important, as the physical, emotional, and practical issues of physical intimacy are now different—and, usually, more difficult.

Yet, survey after survey confirms that most sexually active people are uncomfortable talking about sex with their partners (and their doctors).[2] Specifically, survey participants said they felt more anxious prior to discussing a sexual conflict than a nonsexual one. After your injury, that kind of attitude won't help you, which is why I strongly encourage you and your partner to *read this chapter together*, aloud. This will make having conversations about sex and physical intimacy easier; it doesn't take long for the uncomfortableness to fade away once you begin.

There are four important points to keep in mind as you begin addressing physical intimacy with your partner. But first, let's be clear that physical intimacy and sex are not limited to intercourse; that little three-letter word covers a vast expanse of human behaviors.

1. **Honest communication is essential.** Talking openly with your partner about every aspect of physical intimacy (sexual needs, likes and dislikes, and more) is essential. Good communication is not only expressing your needs but learning how to deliver the message so your partner does not feel burdened, hurt, or misunderstood. This conversation takes two, and needs to be ongoing.

2. **Preservation of pre-injury roles matters greatly to your relationship's viability.** As much as possible, your partner should maintain their role in your relationship from *before* your injury. That's one of many reasons it's important to accept offers of help from family, friends, and neighbors to assist with the multitude of mundane activities of daily living (shopping, errands, appointments, and so on) that can overwhelm your partner. It's difficult to hold on to the romantic and sexual part of your pre-injury life if your partner has become your live-in nurse, therapist, home health aide, and medical liaison.

3. **Romance sets the stage for sexual intimacy.** It's been said that "foreplay begins at the breakfast table." How you treat each other from the time the day begins—the respect, affection, and interest you demonstrate—colors the rest of the day, including the possibility of any sexual interlude. Early in a relationship, romance is a given; over time, many couples seem to forget about it. After an ANI, romance is more important than ever to your relationship, which is, in many ways, a brand-new one. It doesn't take much effort and doesn't even have to cost money; it just needs to be genuine. Even something small, like leaving a love note on the kitchen table, can be deeply meaningful.

4. **Being open to exploring new ways of achieving sexual satisfaction is crucial to your sexual ability and function.** After your injury, don't be reluctant to explore physical intimacy beyond the framework of your pre-injury love life. If none of your doctors or therapists mention it, ask about videos that you and your partner can watch to learn how to be intimate within the restrictions of your injury (these do exist; at my rehab facility, one of my providers gave my wife and me a three-hour-long film to watch. The actors were real couples dealing with ANI limitations). You'll also learn that you can achieve physical pleasure from sensory inputs and sensations that you would not have thought were part of the sexual experience.

There is a recurring theme in the four points outlined above, and that is the ability to be *vulnerable*. Please keep that in mind; it's the cornerstone of long-lasting relationships. Real physical intimacy springs from an *emotional connection*, not merely a physical attraction, and the foundation of that emotional connection is set in place when you allow your vulnerabilities to be seen. Having a deep sense of trust in your partner will allow you the freedom to be vulnerable, which is essential for mutually satisfying sex.

You may not realize it at first, but maintaining physical intimacy with your partner is a profoundly important aspect of your rehabilitation and recovery. So, while there are challenges to overcome, both physically and emotionally, the good news is that there are many treatments for physical sexual enjoyment, including drugs, devices, and surgical procedures that take advantage of existing healthy nerves to enable arousal and physical intimacy. We'll explore these more on pages 112 and 114.

Sexual Function After ANI

Having an ANI does not affect sexual anatomy, but it can cause sexual dysfunction due to problems with motor and sensory function and your body's arousal responses. Renowned sex therapists Masters and Johnson characterized the sexual response with two physiological responses (a systemic increase in blood flow to certain parts of the body and increases in muscle tension), and four successive stages: excitement, plateau, orgasm, and resolution, as detailed in their 1966 book *Human Sexual Response*.[2] After an ANI, there can be changes in how you experience one or more of the four phases that will prevent the next phase from occurring.[3] For some, the phase of excitement (arousal) is markedly decreased due to impaired sensation of the erogenous zones and/or impaired ability of the brain to recognize these sensations due to damage from stroke or TBI.

Sexual arousal includes an increase in heart rate, blood pressure, and breathing, and can include an increase in blood flow to the genitals to prepare your body for sex. For people with vaginas, arousal includes an increase in vaginal lubrication. For people with penises, arousal is signaled by an erection. Arousal happens through two pathways: physical and mental. The reflex pathway (physical) is part of arousal when you are stimulated by sensual touching. Psychogenic arousal (mental) occurs when sensory input alone (seeing, hearing, smelling, or imagining something pleasing to you) turns you on. The brain sends a message via the spinal cord that stimulates vaginal lubrication or develops and maintains an erection.

The brain is the most essential part of sexual arousal. It's responsible for the coordination of the physical response and is considered the "seat of the orgasm." Because orgasm is the desired culmination of sexual arousal for many people, it's the phase that ANI survivors are most concerned about. It's estimated that 50 to 75 percent of people with penises and 50 percent of people with vaginas recover sufficient function to experience orgasm after injury. The orgasm is usually less intense, however, and takes longer to achieve. Although the exact mechanism is unknown, this is likely due to diminished nerve function secondary to damage to the spinal cord and/or the brain.

Sexual Function in Different ANIs

After your injury, you may experience a change in body image, concern about your attractiveness, fear that you will not be able to have intercourse, and worry about the obstacles imposed by your motor deficits (for example, being unable to support yourself in the "top" position).

After SCI, loss of muscle movement, sense of touch, and sexual reflexes is common. The effects on the four stages of the sexual intimacy cycle depend on your level of injury and whether your injury is complete or incomplete. After stroke, the loss of function is usually on one side of the body, leaving the other side intact and able to sense and move normally; the imbalance created, though, can make many movements difficult, especially if you are elderly or have other musculoskeletal problems. After TBI, loss of sensory sharpness and chronic dizziness can present problems; but perhaps more difficult are the behavioral changes that disrupt your ability to engage in social interactions or that derail the phases of the sexual cycle. After TBI and stroke, the nerves to the penis and clitoris are usually preserved, but the ability of the brain to receive sensory feedback and to respond with arousal may be significantly impaired.

Whatever your injury may be, there are a multitude of psychological and physical treatments that can help you maintain your sexual identity and achieve fulfilling sexual experiences.

Changes in Sensation

After your injury, you may experience loss of sensation in the sexual organs that are most sensitive to stimulation—the penis and the clitoris. Both of these organs send and receive sensory and motor information through the nerve roots at the very end of the spinal cord (sacral levels S2–S4). Therefore, if you have spinal cord dysfunction above S2, you probably won't have normal sensation and motor sexual function. There is good news for everyone with ANI: Other areas of your body can be stimulated to provide a sensation that the brain can interpret as sexual. To find these areas, you and your partner should explore and locate your erogenous zones. Some of these are likely to be traditionally sensual areas, such as your nipples, lips, ears, neck, and genital area all the way to mid-thigh. But you may discover entirely new areas that you wouldn't have expected to be pleasurable. People with stroke and TBI are likely to have normal sensation, but the perception by your brain may be decreased, causing difficulty with arousal. Because vision is intact in most people with ANI, watching sexually explicit videos can help to "get going." In addition, stimulation of the penis and clitoris can be performed with aids such as vibrators and vacuum pumps.

Practice makes perfect. Repetitive stimulation of your newfound sensual areas will increase the sensation that your *brain* experiences. This phenomenon—when a nonerogenous zone acquires erogenous characteristics if it is repetitively stimulated during physical intimacy—is another example of neuroplasticity (see chapter 3). Your brain adapts to replace sensual feelings from your penis or clitoris to these new areas.

Bowel and Bladder Involvement

The nerves that exit the spine at S2, S3, and S4, which are necessary for many sexual responses, are also involved in emptying your bowel and bladder. As a result, it's possible for you to have a bowel or bladder "accident" during sexual intimacy, so it's important that you maintain a bowel program (more on this on page 148) and empty your bladder before you begin sexual activity.

Skin Care

Because sexual activity involves rubbing, touching, and squeezing, it's easy to damage skin in areas lacking sensation. As a result, bruising and abrasion of the penis or vulva can occur, especially if lubrication is inadequate. Therefore, lubricants should be used on the genitals prior to sex, if necessary, and both partners should examine their skin after intercourse to be sure that there are no problems. Being aware of potential skin issues is important for a pleasurable and regular sexual experience.

Spasticity

If you have spasticity, you know that certain positions and activities can increase the intensity of the muscle contractions. What you might not know is that the medications that help decrease spasticity may also diminish your sexual drive and your ability to achieve and maintain an erection. This is especially true if you are on multiple medications for spasticity. You may also find that you can actually use spasticity to *enhance* your sexual experience. While spasticity might give you greater strength and enable you to engage in sexual activity for longer periods of time, it alters everyone's sexual response differently.

Medications

You may have noticed that some of your medicines decrease your sexual desire. This is especially true if you are taking more than one medicine that has side effects. After you get home from the hospital and develop a routine, if you notice that your sex drive is greatly diminished, have a conversation with your doctor about your medications. The medications known to affect sexual interest and function include anti-spasticity drugs, some high blood pressure medications (especially thiazide diuretics), a number of heart medicines, and antidepressants.

Autonomic Dysreflexia in Spinal Cord Injury

If your SCI is at T6 or higher, you are at risk for developing autonomic dysreflexia (AD), a condition in which your "involuntary" autonomic nervous system overreacts to external stimuli. AD is characterized by increased blood pressure, increased heart rate, and blurred vision.[4] The nervous system of people with AD overresponds to stimulation that doesn't bother healthy people. This reaction causes a dangerous spike in blood pressure with any type of stimulation below your level of injury. For example, having your nipples stimulated (nerve roots come from T5 and T6) if your injury is at C6–7 (see Figure 2) may cause you to experience AD.

If you experience symptoms of AD, stop sexual activity immediately and wait until the symptoms go away. You can then resume sexual activity, but try a different position. Should the AD recur, speak with your doctor, who may be able to prescribe a medication to decrease the symptoms.

Problems for People with Penises

Erectile Dysfunction (ED) is the inability to get and maintain a firm enough erection for intercourse. Erections are caused by the combination of physical stimulation (reflexogenic) and mental imagery (psychogenic). After ANI, the nerve pathways to and from the brain, as well as the brain itself, may be completely or partially damaged. After SCI, when the injury blocks messages in the brain from reaching their intended destination (T10 through L2 nerves), there will be decreased psychogenic stimulation of erections. Loss of nerve function of S2–S4 will prevent reflexogenic erections. If you've suffered a stroke, you may experience ED as a result of hypertension. Hypertension limits small blood vessels' vasodilation (increase in diameter), which is necessary for an erection. Plus, several hypertension medications also cause ED. After TBI, it is difficult to predict how your injury may affect your ability to maintain an erection, since parts of the brain necessary for psychogenic stimulation of erection may be damaged or dysfunctional.

- **Treatment:** There are many treatments available for ED. Some are as simple as a pill—e.g., Viagra (sildenafil)—that you take prior to intercourse, while others involve devices. You can determine the best treatment options for you by discussing them with your urologist. Insurance usually covers these treatments; your doctor's office can confirm this for you.

Medications

Oral medications for ED include Viagra (sildenafil), Cialis (tadalafil), and Levitra (vardenafil), which are available as pills. Viagra is taken thirty to sixty minutes before engaging in sexual activity, while the others can be taken daily. They all are about 75 percent effective.[5] The major side effect is lowered blood pressure, which decreases the engorgement of blood vessels in the penis. The systemic low blood pressure may make you feel dizzy and uncomfortable. If your ED is a result of low libido, your doctor may prescribe testosterone—but the relationship to CVD is complex. Specifically, persons with low testosterone who replace it to normal levels have less CVD. In contrast, people who take it to high levels have an increase in stroke. Therefore, you need an honest conversation with your doctor regarding benefits and risks.[6] If an oral medication does not enable you to maintain an erection, you should consult with your urologist regarding the options discussed below.

Urethral suppositories are the next drug of choice after oral medication. Alprostadil, which is identical to prostaglandin E1, a substance that occurs naturally in the penis, increases blood flow into the penis, resulting in an erection. It comes as a suppository that is pushed into the tip of the penis, or as a liquid that is injected into the base of the penis.

Other injectable medications include mixtures of drugs that are more potent than alprostadil alone. When injected into the base of the penis, these medications open blood vessels and cause blood to remain in the penis. The most common drugs are papavarine, phentolamine, and alprostadil. Your urologist will prescribe the proper dose of each and the amount to administer. The goal is to give you an erection that lasts between two and four hours. If the erection is poor or short-lasting, you may need to inject more of the drug. Be aware of a potential complication called priapism, which occurs when the blood does not drain from the penis. This results in an erection that lasts longer than four hours, which can cause permanent damage to the penis. Priapism is considered a medical emergency and requires immediate treatment.

Devices

Tension rings are a good choice if you are able to get an erection but unable to maintain it. They're made of rubber or silicone and are placed around the base of the penis, trapping blood in the penis and allowing it to stay erect. They should only be left in place for 30 minutes, because if they are left on too long, they can cause bruising and skin damage.

Vacuum devices, plastic cylinders that are placed over the penis, can be used if you are unable to get an erection and maintain it. The cylinder is attached to a pump that creates a vacuum, which draws blood into the penis, resulting in an erection. You can then place a tension ring at the base of the penis to maintain the erection.

Surgical implants entail the insertion of either flexible rods or inflatable tubes into the penis. This treatment should be a last resort because it has a 10 percent risk of serious complications, most commonly breaking through the skin. Satisfaction among those who use them is high, but if they ever need to be removed, other methods like injections and vacuum devices can't be used due to tissue damage.

Problems for People with Vaginas

Decreased libido. Similar to people with penises, people with vaginas may experience decreased libido or a decreased sexual response. Decreased libido can be caused by antidepressants, such as SSRIs. Testosterone has been shown to increase libido at doses that do not cause changes in the body (such as a deeper voice; more hair, especially on your face; and acne). It should be noted that testosterone has not been approved by the FDA for this purpose. Therefore, you will need to discuss this option with your doctor; if you get a prescription, you will have to have it filled at a special pharmacy.

Vaginal dryness is a problem for many after ANI. During sexual activity, the vagina naturally produces lubrication that helps facilitate sexual activity. For this to happen, both reflexogenic (physical) and psychogenic (mental) stimulation must occur—similar to the process for penile erection. There are a large number of over-the-counter lubricants that can be used prior to and during sexual intercourse; ask your doctor for recommendations. In addition, there are a number of physical stimuli that you and your partner can perform to increase vaginal lubrication, such as oral sex, manual stimulation, and stimulation of other parts of the body such as nipples, ears, and neck. Vaginal dryness can also be treated with a topical or vaginal estrogen cream or patch that stimulates the glands in the vagina to secrete lubricants. Consult with your gynecologist regarding the best approach for you.

Fertility Issues for People with Penises

The fertility rate after ANI varies significantly depending on your age and the severity of your injury. The two major issues are sperm viability and sperm count. The first step in determining your fertility is to see if you can ejaculate on your own. If you're unable to ejaculate or do not have enough viable sperm (determined by a sperm test), the usual treatment is penile vibratory stimulation (PVS) and in vitro fertilization (IVF). PVS involves applying a high-speed vibrator to the head of the penis to trigger ejaculation. The efficacy of PVS to obtain sufficient numbers of viable sperm ranges widely, from 15 to 88 percent, depending on age and severity of injury. If having a family is a priority for you, ask your doctor for a referral to a fertility specialist.

Fertility Issues for People with Vaginas

Unless you've experienced trauma to your reproductive organs, you will typically maintain fertility after your injury. Immediately after injury, you may experience a temporary interruption of your menstrual cycle, which can last up to six months. Once your menstrual cycle resumes, you'll likely be able to become pregnant. If you have difficulty becoming pregnant, you should see your obstetrician, who may refer you to a fertility expert for evaluation and treatment. Other problems that can affect fertility are autonomic dysreflexia (dangerous spike in blood pressure) in SCI, and pituitary hormone insufficiency after TBI, which can affect sexual function, menstruation, and fertility. Should you decide to have a child, discuss with your doctor how pregnancy may affect your injury and your overall health, and if you have the ability to carry a child for nine months.

Here are some of the major issues to consider:

1. Is it likely that pregnancy will increase your disability?

2. What should you do to prepare for changes like swelling of your feet and legs (edema), morning sickness (which may be worse than usual, because of slow stomach emptying due to autonomic nervous system dysfunction), constipation, and urinary tract infections?

3. Will your medications be harmful to your baby? If, for example, you are taking blood thinners for a history of blood clots or cardiovascular disease, it may be necessary to switch to a safer substitute during your pregnancy.

4. Will you need to take medicine for any other health problems? For example, if you have asthma, depression, diabetes, epilepsy, or high blood pressure, you may need to take medications (or change the dose of current drugs) to stay healthy during pregnancy. Your doctor can help you weigh the risks and benefits of each medicine and determine the safest treatment for you and your baby.

5. What over-the-counter medications are safe to take during pregnancy? Be careful and ask your obstetrician. For example, supplements like feverfew, ginseng, kava, licorice, sage, St. John's wort, senna, white peony, and large doses of vitamin A may cause harm to the developing baby.

These last four chapters have focused on regaining your health, both mentally and physically. While many of the suggested therapies do not require drugs or devices, an equal number involve medications. Unfortunately, medications come with side effects, and the more you take, the more likely that two or more will interact to cause harmful side effects. Therefore, many people look for ways to heal themselves in other ways. In the next chapter, you'll learn about some different approaches derived from traditional Eastern medicine.

Everything You Need to Know

Physical intimacy is an emotional nutrient, absolutely essential to the viability of a long-term loving partnership. After your injury, your ability for sexual relations with your partner may change a little or a lot. The bedrock of a satisfying, genuine, and long-lasting physically intimate relationship is open, honest, and respectful communication. Here's what you and your partner need to know:

1. It's necessary to talk to each other about sex, and to be aware that it is not going to be a one-time conversation.

2. Romance is vital to build and maintain an authentic and satisfying lifelong physical and sexual intimacy with your partner.

3. Your partner should try to maintain their pre-injury role in the relationship as much as possible. Becoming the default full-time caregiver can damage your relationship.

4. Be creative in your exploration of the new boundaries of your sexual abilities and needs.

5. Remember that your biggest, most powerful sexual organ is your brain.

6. Your libido may decrease due to brain damage. Because of decreased sensation in motor innervation, you may experience erectile or clitoral dysfunction. For people with vaginas, decreased vaginal lubrication may require the use of lubricants.

7. Fertility may become a problem because of hormonal, sensory, motor, and autonomic nervous system dysfunction. See a fertility expert if this applies to you.

8

East Meets West

*How to Use Modern Western Medicine and
Traditional Eastern Medicine to Heal
and Enjoy a Better Quality of Life*

I'M A BOARD-CERTIFIED CARDIOLOGIST and a biomedical scientist. From my medical training and experience as a doctor, I hold a long-standing faith in the value of what we call Western medicine. But, since my spinal cord injury, I've learned that there are tremendous benefits to be found in Eastern (or Asian) medicine and complementary medicines and therapies.

The story behind my knowledge of Eastern medicine is one of friendship, compassion, and medical brilliance. It begins with Dr. Guoyong Yin, an orthopedic surgeon from Nanjing, China, who was a research fellow in my laboratory. In 2010, Dr. Yin introduced me to Dr. Jianan Li, the President of the Zhongshan Rehabilitation Hospital in Nanjing, China. Dr. Li told me that I had made an excellent recovery, but he thought that I could make much more progress if I devoted more time to rehabilitation and less time to being a CEO. He offered me the opportunity to stay in Nanjing for three to six months to perform intense rehabilitation for six hours daily. After I stepped down as CEO, Dr. Li and I discussed a rehab program, and he arranged for me to stay for six weeks in the fall of 2017.

My time there was the most profound healing experience to date. The rehabilitation approach was what we call integrative medicine: Western medicine combined with complementary medicine. In my case, traditional Chinese medicine (TCM) was the complementary approach.[1] The success of this approach involves the following:

• A holistic understanding of you as a person and a focus on using your strengths to improve function through complementary therapies, especially massage and acupuncture

- The technique of improving *one* movement and the muscles necessary for that movement, which translates into significant improvements in other movements and muscles

- An approach that focuses on improving physical function, especially walking, to improve sensation

The Chinese Diet

It should be noted that significant changes in my diet occurred while I was in China, most notably an increase in fish consumption and a decrease in processed carbohydrates (bread, cereal, pasta, and other baked goods). These changes altered the composition of my gut microbiome (the bacteria that live in the colon and are responsible for the strength of the immune system), which led to a number of beneficial effects on my health.

The Chinese diet's role in optimal health became widely known in 2006 after the publication of *The China Study*,[2] by T. Colin Campbell and Thomas M. Campbell (updated in 2016[3]). From huge studies conducted in China and Taiwan, they concluded that the typical American diet had too much protein and fat. They emphasize following a whole-food plant-based diet, with no processed foods or supplements. Although it advocates for a predominantly plant-based diet, *The China Study* also recommends seafood as an excellent source of protein. Significant research supports that advice; omega-3 fatty acids found in wild-caught ocean-dwelling fish are beneficial to the heart and brain.[4] A recent randomized trial showed, in patients with elevated triglyceride levels, the risk of CVD events was significantly lower among those who received 2 g of icosapent ethyl, a purified fish oil.[5] Plus, research shows that meat-derived proteins undergo metabolism in the gut that produces toxic products (e.g., trimethylamine N-oxide, TMAO) that can harm some of the body's organs, especially blood vessels in the heart and brain.[6]

Integrative Medicine

Integrative medicine refers to the use of conventional Western medicine *in tandem* with complementary medicine. This is different from complementary and alternative medicine (CAM), which includes use of alternative medicine *in place of* Western medicine. Examples of complementary medicine include acupuncture, acupressure, Ayurveda, aromatherapy, massage, and meditation.[7] Examples of alternative medicine include many elements of traditional Chinese medicine (TCM), such as mixtures of various plant and animal materials specific to that tradition given as pills, tinctures, creams, and other topical formulations. I've found the most success in combining Western conventional medicine with complementary medicine, but you may want to experiment to see what works best for you.

The fact that more than 50 percent of Americans now use some type of CAM on a routine basis indicates just how mainstream Eastern medicine has become in the US.[8] And, within the ANI population, the rate of CAM use is even *higher* than in the general population.[9] So, if this is all new to you, be assured that many others find benefit from these approaches to healing.

Eastern and Western Philosophies

The philosophy of TCM assumes that the forces, which govern the cycles of change in the external world are duplicated within our bodies and minds. TCM emphasizes the importance of understanding the laws of nature and abiding by these laws rather than resisting them. The human body is regarded as a microcosmic reflection of the universe. The goal of TCM is to maintain the body's harmonious balance both internally and in relation to our environment.

TCM focuses on mechanisms in the human body that regulate function. Western philosophy approximates Eastern philosophy in its approach to the mind, which requires two actions of faith. First, the mind is the seat of thought that arises from the brain's activity. The development of functional MRI has enabled us to see which parts of the brain become active when you think. Simple thoughts, like *move my finger*, activate a small amount of the motor cortex that controls the nerves in your hands. More profound thinking, especially with an emotional component, activates many more areas of the brain. Second, the mind exists outside of sensory perception. This means that there's no physical manifestation of the brain that you can sense (headaches don't count). The mind represents the highest level of human intellect and is the source of questions regarding the existence of mankind and the universe. This has led to an experimental approach to understanding the forces that control our world, which can be used to control the body's interactions with the world. Over the last 150 years, medicine has been profoundly affected by an approach in which each disease is reduced to a single cause that may be treated with a single drug. A classic example is streptococcal pneumonia, for which treatment with penicillin dramatically improved recovery from what had previously been a fatal illness.

Traditional Chinese Medicine (TCM)

Eastern medicine, particularly TCM, observes and describes the functions of the body based on the harmony between humans and nature, as exemplified by the concept of qi. The three most important concepts in TCM are qi, yin/yang, and five elements.

- **Qi is frequently translated as *vital energy*.** It is believed that it permeates all things, can assume different forms, and travels through channels (or meridians) in the body. When a person's qi is described as stagnant, depleted, collapsed, or rebellious, TCM is used to restore positive energy. A skilled TCM practitioner determines the nature of a patient's problem and prescribes acupuncture, herbal medicines, massage, meditation, and other therapies to restore balance and maximize qi.

- **Yin and yang are complementary opposites**—light and dark, good and bad, noisy and quiet, strong and weak, and so on—that describe all things in nature. Yin represents the more material, dense states of matter, while yang represents the immaterial, more rarefied states of matter. TCM therapies seek to restore the balance of yin and yang.

- **Five elements (wood, water, fire, earth, and metal)**, along with yin and yang, form the basis of Chinese medical theory. Each of these elements can generate or counteract another element. Most vital organs, acupuncture meridians, and emotions are assigned an element, providing a global description of the person's overall health as measured by the strength and symmetry of their qi.

Traditional Chinese Medicine (TCM) Therapies for ANI

Acupuncture, a key component of TCM, involves the insertion of thin, sterile metal needles into specific locations (acupoints) located on fourteen main energy channels (meridians) distributed throughout the body.[10] These meridians are associated with specific organs, like the liver (Figure 15).

There are fourteen acupoints in the liver meridian, which extends from the groin to the liver, and then from the liver to the nipple, and ultimately to the right ear.

Acupuncture treatments are customized for each individual, meaning that two patients with the same injury will often receive different treatments. I found that acupuncture was effective for pain relief of my right arm and shoulder, which had experienced complex regional pain syndrome (CRPS) for many years. Clinical studies have shown that acupuncture is useful for four chronic pain conditions: back and neck pain, osteoarthritis, chronic headache, and shoulder pain.[11] You may also choose to seek out acupuncture if you have CRPS, neuropathic pain, and problems with bladder and bowel function.

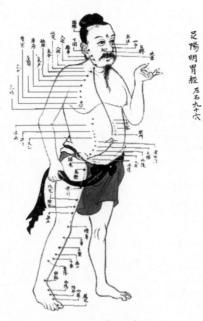

Figure 15. Diagram of Meridians

Massage

The two major effects of massage that are consistent in clinical trials are a decrease in pain and a decrease in muscle soreness after exercise. The most likely mechanism for decreasing pain is based on the gate control theory, which states that pressure signals are transmitted faster than pain signals, thus closing the pathway for pain signals to the brain.[12] The decrease in muscle soreness is probably due to the ability of massage to increase flow through arteries, veins, and lymphatics. Increased blood and lymphatic flow should reduce inflammation, according to multiple reviews of massage clinical trials, which show decreased biomarkers of muscle damage and inflammation.[13] The utility of massage for pain reduction may be greater with some massage techniques, especially those that increase blood flow, and hence decrease the stimuli for inflammation. I recommend that you try several types of massage and several practitioners to find the combination that works best for you.

The most common styles of massage include the following:

- Pressure-point techniques (also referred to as shiatsu, trigger point, and acupressure), which most closely resemble the types of massage found in China. A massage technique that is popular in TCM but little known in the US is tui na. Tui na uses rapid tapping with the thumb to loosen tendons and muscles, as well as kneading, rolling, pressing, and rubbing. There are other types of massage that you can try, each with its own "style."

- Swedish massage (long, gliding strokes; kneading)

- Deep-tissue massage (such as Rolfing and Hellerwork)

- Craniosacral therapy (gentle touch to the joints of the skull)

- Neuromuscular massage (digital pressure and friction to release areas of strain in a muscle)

I've found massage to be the *most* valuable complementary therapy—so much so that I go twice weekly for a one-hour session. Pressure-point massage techniques work best for me, and my home health aides use an electric massage tool to relax my shoulders and arms during the day and before I go to bed.

The massage therapist is frequently more important than the type of massage. Most states have license or certificate programs that establish a certain level of knowledge and expertise, and I encourage you to check the therapist's credentials. Ask the massage therapist to explain the anatomy of your problem and their approach to it. People with ANI have many of the same problems as nondisabled people, so you need not necessarily seek out a specialist—an excellent massage therapist will be just as excellent for you.

Meditation and Mindfulness

Meditation and mindfulness have origins in multiple medical philosophies and are now used universally (see chapter 4 for more). Clinical trials show that both meditation and mindfulness promote overall health by increasing calmness and reducing stress (see chapter 2). These techniques can benefit everyone—whether you're healthy, injured, or ill. And if you're living with an injury, they can be a powerful part of your healing and improving your quality of life.

Mindfulness is the practice of maintaining complete awareness of one's thoughts, emotions, and experiences on a moment-to-moment basis. It's a simple tool you can use throughout your day. Mindfulness promotes clear thinking, compassion, and open-mindedness. Multiple studies show significant benefits of mindfulness to decrease chronic pain.[14] Among possible mechanisms are greater perceived control of pain that results from a decreased emotional response to pain.[15] An easy approach to mindfulness is the three-element practice of "Pause, Presence, Proceed" popularized by the University of Wisconsin.[16]

Pause: Stop and take a breath.

Presence: Make yourself aware of what is happening in your environment, focusing on body sensations, thoughts, and emotions.

Proceed: Communicate with those around you using compassion and positive words to address the issues that you became aware of while practicing presence.

Meditation involves engaging in mental exercise for the purpose of reaching a heightened level of awareness. While there are many forms of meditation (religious, self-realization, transcendental, Tibetan Buddhism, and Zen Buddhism, among others), practices share many common features, so your choice will be determined by your relationship with your teacher and/or which meditation practices you find most beneficial. Meditation has myriad health benefits, especially for cardiovascular health.[17] It has been shown to lower blood pressure, decrease biomarkers associated with heart attacks, improve cardiac function related to coronary artery disease, and provide positive effects on biopsychosocial measures: biological (physical and mental health), psychological (mood, personality and behavior), and social (culture, family and socioeconomic).[18]

The process of starting meditation has an easy mnemonic[19]: **SOLAR.**

Stop: Find a quiet place where you will not be disturbed for at least five minutes; pause and begin.

Observe: Pay attention to what is happening moment by moment.

Let it be: Let everything be as it is without reacting to it or trying to change it.

And Return: Come back to the present moment, remembering to pause, breathe, and feel.

My Meditation Practice

I meditate every morning before I get up to start the day. I usually wake at 7:00, and my home health aide comes in at 7:15, so I have fifteen minutes to meditate and then perform a few physical exercises. Once I'm fully awake, I take a survey of my entire body, feeling how all of my limbs are lined up and making sure that I'm in a comfortable position. Then I imagine myself in a state of complete relaxation, almost floating. At the rehab facility, I would do this outdoors, reclined in my wheelchair. I would watch the clouds float by in the sky, feel the wind against my face, and listen to the sound of the leaves moving in the trees. Now, I watch the trees and sky through our big bedroom window and listen to the sounds of the wind and my house. I focus on breathing and the phrase *let it be*, because I find this relaxes me the most. I stop when my inner clock lets me know that seven or eight minutes have gone by. This seemingly simple daily practice allows me to begin my day with a sense of relaxation and clarity. You may be thinking, *I don't have time for that*, but I assure you, you do. And it will be time well spent. Once meditation becomes a habit, you won't want to skip it.

Yoga and Tai Chi: Mind/Body Therapies

In the United States, yoga is by far the most widely practiced of the Eastern mind/body practices. Modern yoga, which originated in India, has three main components: postures/poses (asanas), breath control (pranayama), and meditation (samyama). Poses range from simple stretching positions to more complicated, difficult postures. Breath control is slow, deep, diaphragmatic breathing that helps you achieve a state of relaxation.

There are many reasons why people practice yoga, but for the vast majority, it's simply one part of a healthy lifestyle. Many studies have investigated the health benefits associated with yoga. Most randomized controlled studies that compare yoga with no intervention or treatment as usual find statistically significant benefits in several domains. These include physical health, decreased stress, improved quality of life, reduced pain, and improvement in symptoms of many diseases. However, when compared to exercise, the benefits from yoga are about the same, suggesting that you should choose whichever activity you enjoy more. In terms of pain, there's strong evidence that yoga can decrease pain, especially low back pain.[20] Despite the limitations in physical movement associated with ANI, yoga can be an important component of rehabilitation. The key is to use modified poses and props, as described in Iyengar yoga, like pillows, blankets, and bolsters to enable therapeutic yoga exercise.

Overall, the studies of yoga for ANI show improvements in strength, flexibility, and relaxation.[21] However, for neuropathic pain, there are limited data on the use and effectiveness of yoga. Matthew Sanford, a noted yoga teacher and person with an SCI, says that performing yoga reunites the mind-body connection and, in so doing, decreases pain, including neuropathic pain.[22] It should be noted, however, that some of the yoga positions are quite difficult for ANI survivors to perform and may cause injuries, especially to muscles and ligaments. Therefore, I recommend that you start with Iyengar yoga.[23] Check with your therapy team about which poses would be safe for you to try.

Tai chi involves dancelike movement and martial arts movement in conjunction with mindfulness. There are many styles of tai chi, just like yoga, so they both have universal appeal. Both activities occur in classes and so provide an opportunity for significant social interaction. Which activity you choose is a personal preference (and you can do both if you want to!).

Herbs and Supplements

Over the last ten years, the most commonly used CAM therapies have been herbal and dietary supplements, with expenditures of $12.8 billion for nonvitamin, nonmineral natural products.[24] There are hundreds of commonly used herbs derived from traditional Chinese medicine. They're often available in grocery stores, pharmacies, and health food stores; common herbs include ginseng, ginkgo, wolfberry, astragalus, cinnamon, curcumin, ephedra, ginger, peony, and salvia. Unfortunately, some of these natural products can be unhealthy, especially at higher doses. For most CAM medicines, efficacy and toxicity are based on traditional knowledge rather than laboratory analysis. Because the amounts of active chemicals are often not listed on the medicine bottles, and there's no way to know the exact preparation, it's difficult to take the same dose each time and expect the same effect. This is particularly problematic if you switch from one manufacturer to another; the same CAM herb or supplement from a different source might have twice as much active ingredient per pill, leading to a toxic overdose.

Medicines derived from plants are used in Western medicine as well, and many have been with us a long time; aspirin was originally found in the bark of willow trees, and the first statin drug to lower cholesterol was found in rice. Unfortunately, using TCM medications can place you at substantial risk for harm, because of poor quality control of ingredients and manufacturing. Also, there are few clinical trials that show significant benefit compared to placebo. For these reasons, I don't recommend TCM supplements. You may find that your doctor can guide you in a careful use of them. If so, the subject is worthy of a thorough discussion.

––––––

Everything You Need to Know

Thoughtful integration of aspects of traditional Eastern medicine with Western medicine have greatly enhanced my recovery. As you explore the various options available to you, here's what you need to know:

- Integrative Medicine (the combination of Western medicine with traditional Eastern medicine/therapies) offers many benefits as you continue your recovery.

- Several traditional Chinese medicine (TCM) treatments are known to benefit health, most notably acupuncture, massage, and tai chi. All can decrease pain and promote nerve and muscle recovery.

- Adopting the Chinese diet, which emphasizes a whole-food plant-based diet and decreased animal protein (except for seafood) can improve your overall health.

- Meditation and mindfulness are practices that promote clear thinking, compassion, and physical relaxation—all beneficial as you work through rehabilitation therapies.

- Yoga has been shown to decrease pain, especially lower back pain.

- There are hundreds of herbs and supplements in the United States, many of which are derived from traditional Chinese medicine. Because there is no standardization of ingredients and frequently no quality control in manufacturing, they pose a substantial risk for harm, so talk to your doctor before use.

PART 3

Preventing and Treating the Most Common Medical Problems

Urinary Tract and
Bladder Health

I F YOU HAD ASKED me, before I was living with my disability, which organ would give me the greatest difficulty, I would have said my brain (because the medications make people sleepy and forgetful) or my arms and legs (because they were paralyzed). I was surprised to find that my bladder has actually given me the most problems, including but not limited to urinary tract infections (UTIs). In fact, this is true for almost everyone with an SCI and for many people after stroke.

The urogenital tract (Figure 16) starts at the kidneys, which filter the blood and create urine. Urine flows to the bladder via tubes called the ureters and into the bladder. As the bladder fills up and descends, it sends a signal to the brain that it is time to empty. When you are ready to go to the bathroom, the external sphincter of the urethra opens, allowing urine to pass. In people with penises, the urethra passes through the prostate, which frequently enlarges and squeezes the urethra, causing difficulty in passing urine. The urethra then goes through the penis. In people with vaginas, there is no prostate and a much shorter urethra, with an opening in the vulva.

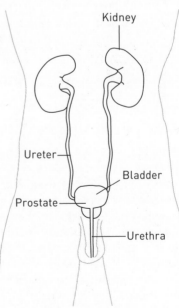

Figure 16. Male urinary tract anatomy

A Disaster Waiting to Happen

It turns out that when you no longer have control of your bladder, urine either doesn't come out when you want it to (neurogenic bladder) or comes out when you don't expect it (incontinent bladder). In both situations, urine is likely to come in contact with bacteria in your groin, which can swim up into your bladder. Here, bacteria find a warm, nutrient-rich environment, so they grow quickly—the perfect scenario for infection.

In my case, this lack of control can mean not only UTIs but also embarrassing leaks around the tube site (I've found all kinds of tactics to avoid that, but urine can leak down my groin, wetting my underwear, shirt, pants, and finally, my wheelchair cushion). If you're particularly unfortunate, the urine will drip onto your wheelchair or, even worse, onto the floor (usually carpeted!).

Neurogenic Bladder

Neurogenic bladder describes a number of urinary conditions in people who lack bladder control due to a brain, spinal cord, or peripheral nerve problem. Even if you suffered from neurogenic bladder at the time of your hospitalization, you'll likely recover if your injury was a stroke or TBI. SCI survivors are the most likely to experience chronic neurogenic bladder, although some stroke patients will as well. People with chronic neurogenic bladder frequently have some of these symptoms: problems starting to urinate or emptying their bladder, frequent urination in small amounts, incontinence due to both sudden spasms and a constant leak, and inability to sense how full their bladder is.

SCI-Specific Urinary Problems

After SCI, you may experience "spastic bladder" or "flaccid bladder."
A spastic bladder fills with urine, and a reflex automatically triggers it to empty. Since you don't know when the bladder will empty, sudden leakage can occur. With a flaccid bladder, the reflexes of the bladder muscles are absent. You can't feel when the bladder is full, so it can become stretched (or overdistended) beyond its normal capacity, causing urine to back up through the ureters into the kidneys. This chronic reflux is damaging to the kidneys and, over time, can cause kidney failure. Both spastic and flaccid bladders can be treated with continuous bladder drainage. This can be accomplished using Foley catheters (see page 133) for short periods of time or suprapubic tubes (see page 136) for long-term treatment.

Urinary Tract Problems and Treatments

Keep in mind that as we get older, problems that impair bladder function increase in everyone, disabled or not. In people with penises, the most common problem is enlargement of the prostate (benign prostatic hypertrophy, or BPH), which then squeezes the urethra (Figure 16), making it difficult to urinate and necessitating frequent trips to the bathroom. In people with vaginas, the pelvic floor that keeps the bladder and its opening (sphincter) tight can become weak, making incontinence common. Because these changes are frequently part of the aging process, bladder management can be even more difficult as you get older. But there are a variety of treatments to combat these issues.

Bladder Management

There are several short- and long-term solutions for treating bladder dysfunction. After my accident, when I was in the intensive care unit, my bladder was drained continuously using a Foley catheter, a sterile tube inserted into the urethra (Figure 17). The Foley catheter is a temporary, short-term solution due to its size and the fact that it can introduce harmful bacteria into the urethra. It can also irritate and even damage the urinary tract, especially in people with penises.

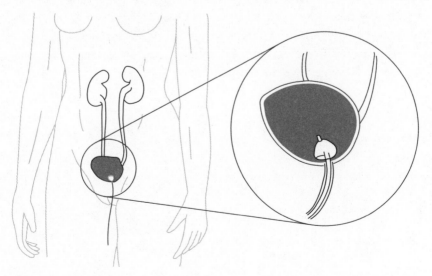

Figure 17. Foley catheter

The long-term solutions to bladder management share three goals: 1) to make you as independent as possible, 2) to control *when* you urinate, and 3) to prevent urinary tract infections (UTIs) and kidney damage. The most common long-term solutions are Credé and Valsalva, self-catheterization, suprapubic tube, indwelling Foley catheter, and condom catheter.

Credé and Valsalva: In people with near-normal bladder function, it can be difficult to initiate urination because the external urethral sphincter won't open. A simple solution is to increase the pressure in the bladder that forces the sphincter to open. The most common technique is called Credé's maneuver, in which pressure is put on the abdomen below the navel to push on the bladder. The pressure can be further increased by performing a Valsalva maneuver, in which you inhale a large breath and then bear down as if having a bowel movement. The increased downward pressure forces the sphincter to open, but be careful: Too much pressure can cause sphincter damage and incontinence.

Self-catheterization: Self-catheterization involves manually inserting a sterile tube through the urethra and into the bladder (Figure 18A & B). Depending on your fluid intake, you'll have to do this four to six times daily. You need to be able to sense bladder fullness, and/or regulate fluid intake so that the bladder does not overdistend. If there's too much urine in the bladder, pressure can be transmitted up through the ureters to the kidneys, eventually resulting in kidney damage. Self-catheterization requires good manual dexterity to ensure that the catheter enters the urethra properly and to maintain tube sterility during the process so as not to introduce bacteria into the bladder. Recent advances in catheter design have resulted in self-lubricating catheters that contain their

A 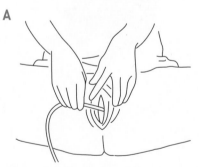 B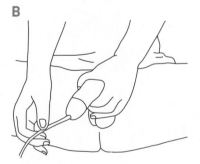

Figure 18. Self catheterization

own drainage bag and can be used with only one hand. Of course, they cost quite a bit more than the basic catheters. The major advantages of self-catheterization are independence, cosmetic appearance, and no permanent object (catheter) in the bladder. A permanent catheter, like the Foley or suprapubic tube, will become colonized with bacteria over time, which may cause UTIs.

Reflex voiding—condom catheter: Reflex voiding occurs when the bladder contracts involuntarily, even when it's not full. To manage this, condom catheters, or external catheters, can be worn on the penis like a condom (Figure 19A & B). These are much less invasive than internal catheters, like Foley catheters, which must be inserted into the bladder. The major advantage of condom catheters is convenience, since a leg bag can be used to collect urine continuously (Figure 19B). The biggest advantage of a condom catheter is that incontinence won't interfere with sleep; the major disadvantage is irritation of the penis, which can be minimized by appropriate sizing of the condom catheter, maintaining excellent hygiene, and moisturizing the skin. However, sometimes the skin on the penis becomes so damaged that it cannot tolerate the condom catheter. If a condom catheter cannot be used due to breakdown of penis skin, absorbent underwear must be worn until the skin recovers. This is unpleasant in terms of comfort and smell.

A

B

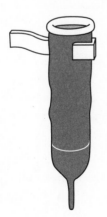
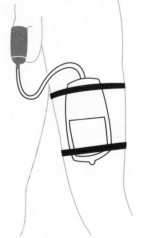

Figure 19. Condom catheter

Suprapubic tube (SPT): Insertion of an SPT requires a small surgery in which a tunnel is made from just below the navel to the bladder, and a catheter is passed into the bladder (Figure 20). Similar to a Foley catheter, it continuously drains the bladder. It's connected to a leg bag that can hold 1 to 2 liters (about 1 to 2 quarts) of urine, depending on the size you need. SPT has several advantages over both an indwelling urethral catheter and self-catheterization. Since it doesn't

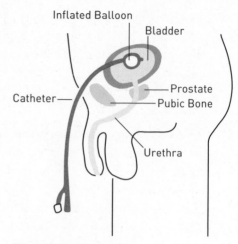

Figure 20. Suprapubic tube

require sterile technique, it can be used by people with poor dexterity; you either unscrew a tip or flip a clamp to let the urine drain out. Compared to the Foley catheter, the SPT cannot damage the urethra; it's less likely to get kinked or blocked, since the catheter is wider; everyone can use it; and it doesn't interfere with sex. The SPT can be easily removed if bladder function improves; once the catheter is removed, the tunnel closes in a few days. There's no restriction on fluid intake, and if your urine output varies significantly over the course of the day, there's no risk of bladder distension and subsequent kidney damage. The cost of SPT is comparable to self-catheterization as long as the collection bags are changed every seven to fourteen days and sterilized daily with bleach.

There are, however, more complications with SPT than with self-catheterization. The two major problems are bladder or kidney stones, and an increased risk for bladder cancer (especially if using the SPT for more than ten years). Bladder stones occur in at least 10 percent of people with SPTs.[1] They are problematic because they can plug the catheter, shorten the duration of its use, cause more bladder spasticity and leaks, and serve as additional objects for bacteria to colonize.

Surgical procedures: There are several surgical procedures that can be considered as alternatives to SPT. Among these, the Mitrofanoff procedure (Mitrofanoff appendicovesicostomy) involves connecting the navel to the bladder using the appendix as a conduit. It's most commonly performed as an elective procedure for people with vaginas, because it avoids contamination from bacteria in the vagina, is easier than self-catheterization, is cosmetically appealing, and doesn't interfere with sex. The major disadvantage is that it requires surgery, which has a higher risk of complications than SPT surgery.

Drug treatments: There are a number of drugs that can improve bladder function, but many of them have undesirable side effects: constipation, dry mouth, and blood pressure increases or decreases. Drugs that inhibit bladder spasticity include anticholinergic drugs (e.g., oxybutynin, solifenacin, tolterodine, and fesoterodine), and mirabegron, a beta 3-adrenoceptor agonist with fewer side effects than anticholinergics—notably, less dry mouth and constipation. These medications decrease bladder tone and suppress bladder spasms, thereby reducing urinary frequency and incontinence.

More invasive and expensive therapies are usually reserved for people who are intolerant to drug therapy. Botulinum toxin (Botox) can be injected into the bladder to relax the muscle and lessen spasticity by inhibiting the nerve transmitter acetylcholine. A comprehensive analysis of nineteen trials showed significant decreases in urgency, bladder spasms, and leakage that were better than medications.[2] The toxin lasts for six to twelve months and has no systemic side effects, making it particularly safe and effective, though it increases the risk for UTIs and urinary retention.

Devices: Electrical stimulation of nerves that supply the bladder to control bladder spasticity is a rapidly evolving technology. The most common approach is sacral neuromodulation, in which an electrode is placed

My History of UTIs

I used a Foley catheter for the first six weeks after my injury, but I developed a UTI and had blood in my urine. Because my injury was high in the cervical spine, the strength and dexterity of my hands and arms were limited. I couldn't self-catheterize, so I chose a suprapubic tube (SPT), which worked quite well, at first. I had only one UTI, which was readily treated with antibiotics. Then, after two years of use, I began to develop leaks around the SPT that occurred at the most inopportune times. In the middle of an important meeting, I would look down and see an expanding area of my pants becoming darker. I would smell an odor that resembled apple cider, which indicated that urine was flowing around the SPT and into my pants. Sometimes, it was wicked up by my undershirt and dress shirt, leaving a visible yellowish-brown stain. With the help of my urologist, we battled the problem on two fronts: prevention and defense.

into the lower spine and connected to an electrical stimulation device. The current approved FDA devices are the Axonics and InterStim. But these devices have not been extensively used in people with ANI, so I wouldn't recommend them at this time. I believe that in the future, there will be significantly better devices to restore bladder function.

UTI and Bladder Spasm Prevention and Defense

The major goals of prevention are to limit bladder spasms and UTIs. A common cause of leaks for those using SPT is bladder spasms. These occur more commonly in people with indwelling catheters, because the bladder shrinks and the muscle becomes irritable. This is worsened by UTIs, which make the bladder even more spastic. The medical solution is drugs (such as oxybutynin) that inhibit spasticity. These drugs have numerous side effects; the most notable of which are dry mouth, constipation, and drowsiness.

The first line of defense is absorbent padding, such as disposable absorbent briefs (such as Depend), which are commonly used for people with vaginas. But briefs can be bulky in those with penises, making your pants fit poorly. They can also make you hot, sweaty, and uncomfortable. Instead, people with penises may choose to use an abdominal barrier pad, which is absorbent on one side and water-resistant on the other, taped into their underwear. The problem with this solution is that the pad can absorb only a small amount of urine before the urine finds a way to flow down below the pad and onto your clothes.

If you're experiencing frequent leaks and/or UTIs, use this chapter to help you identify the problems that give rise to them, and develop solutions. Each person is unique, so whatever system works best for you is what matters.

Urinary Tract Infections (UTIs)

Diagnosis: You may be surprised to read that UTI diagnosis can be difficult—even more so if you have an indwelling catheter. The catheter constantly irritates the bladder, causing white blood cells to accumulate, and over time, the bladder becomes colonized with bacteria. In people with normal bladder function, the presence of white blood cells and bacteria, accompanied by frequent urination (with urgency) is typical of a UTI. In people with ANI, however, these things are present when there is *no* UTI. The question, then, is what *are* symptoms of a UTI that requires treatment in people with ANI?

Most infections increase body temperature, but UTIs frequently don't, especially in older people. Symptoms may include pain in the lower abdomen, increased spasticity, feeling sick, fatigue, headache, incontinence, and urgency. The first time I had a UTI after my injury, I knew something was wrong—I was incredibly cold, my muscles hurt, and my arms and hands were flexed inward (assuming an almost fetal position). When I have a UTI, I can tell from three changes in my urine, which are common in most people with UTIs. First, my urine becomes cloudy; when I hold a piece of printed paper behind the urine container (I use a clear container), I can't read the words. Second, it begins to smell bad, like rotten meat. Third, I experience bladder spasms that result in urine leaking around my SPT site. After two or three UTIs, you'll learn to recognize your symptoms, too. If these symptoms don't resolve within twenty-four hours, ask your doctor to order a urinalysis and a urine culture to determine which bacteria are present and what antibiotics you'll need.

Treatment: Once a UTI has been diagnosed, there are two highly effective treatments: antibiotics and forcing fluids. *If you don't have a catheter*, your doctor may prescribe antibiotics if you show systemic signs of UTI (fever, spasticity, pain, and fatigue). The antibiotics must be proven by laboratory testing to kill the bacteria, and you'll need to drink at *least* two quarts of water and other fluids every day to help "wash out" the bacteria.

If you have a catheter (Foley or SPT), it's best to avoid antibiotics unless you have significant systemic signs. The catheter will almost always contain bacteria that can't be killed, so using antibiotics will ultimately lead to dangerous drug-resistant bacteria in your catheter.

So what can you do? There are no good clinical studies to guide us, but there are several treatments I and many others have found effective. The safest is to increase fluid intake so that the volume of urine increases. My mantra for this treatment is *the more the flow, the less they grow.* When you have an infection, the bacteria attach themselves to your bladder wall and build a covering called a biofilm, which protects them from patrolling white blood cells. But when there's a large volume of urine flow, the bacteria can't build their biofilm, and they are flushed out of the bladder. Another approach is to lower the pH of your urine (acidification), which makes it difficult for the bacteria to live and grow. There are many suggested remedies, but I have found that using a dilute form of bleach, clorpactin, is very effective when I have a UTI. It is infused into my bladder through the SPT and stays there for two treatments of two minutes. Also, lowering your pH with vitamin C and methenamine hippurate or methenamine mandelate (my preference), can be effective as prevention in the long term. Some people use a powerful antibiotic (like gentamicin) in saline solution to wash their bladder. (This treatment was never effective for me.)

If you have bladder stones, the best treatment is to dissolve the stones. Renacidin—a combination of citric acid, glucono-delta-lactone, and magnesium carbonate—is often prescribed as a solution of 50 ml, which is infused through the tube and drained after forty-five minutes. It must be used three to four times daily for several days to dissolve the stones. If the stones are too large, it won't work, and your urologist will have to physically remove the stones using a special endoscope.

Prevention of UTIs

Frequent UTIs can be extremely frustrating. If left untreated, they can spread to the kidneys and even to the bloodstream, causing an infection called sepsis; it's serious, and it requires hospitalization and intravenous antibiotics. For all these reasons, *prevention* should be a major focus of your everyday life.

Treat Fatigue and Stress: Unfortunately, fatigue and stress are prevalent in many of us, and they make you more susceptible to UTIs. Fatigue is slightly easier to address. You'll need to get enough sleep for your body to heal (at *least* seven hours and preferably eight each night). And don't overdo it when working or playing. When you begin to feel tired, it's time to stop and rest. Stress is much more difficult to treat because we don't always recognize when we're experiencing it. The good news is that the same methods that increase your awareness of stress also help you reduce stress: self-awareness, mindfulness, and meditation (see chapter 8).

Take D-mannose: One of the most common bacteria that cause UTIs is *Escherichia coli* (*E. coli*), which is found in stool. *E. coli* infects the bladder by binding to the epithelial cells that line the bladder. Because the binding site looks like D-mannose (a sugar, like glucose), the idea is to trick the *E. coli* to bind to the D-mannose and then be flushed out with the urine. Because D-mannose is specific for bacteria and is 100 percent excreted in the urine, it has almost no side effects. D-mannose is taken as 1 g twice daily, either dissolved in a powder or as a pill by mouth.

Practice good dental hygiene: If you have periodontitis (infection of the gums), your gums shed bacteria that enter the bloodstream. During routine flossing and hygiene, this bacteria shedding can increase significantly. The bacteria travel through the bloodstream to the kidneys and then are excreted in the urine. Meticulous attention to dental hygiene to prevent and cure periodontitis is very important to decrease bacteria in the bladder.

Increase fluid intake: A very simple approach to preventing UTIs is to increase flow through the bladder. Try to drink eight 8-ounce glasses of liquid every day. This regimen is simple to remember and easy if you have continuous drainage of your bladder by Foley, SPT, or condom catheter. If you use self-catheterization, it's inconvenient to catheterize more than three or four times per day, so most people will limit fluid intake, especially after dinner. Because you have no permanent catheter for bacteria to attach to and grow, it's less important for you to increase urine flow.

Take methenamine hippurate or methenamine mandelate and vitamin C: Acidic urine (low pH) prevents bacterial growth. Methenamine, when taken with vitamin C, lowers urine pH. It is generally well tolerated, except for mild abdominal cramps; many people (myself included) have found it to be beneficial. You can do an empirical trial yourself: Count the number of UTIs you have over six months while taking 500 mg methenamine plus 1,000 mg vitamin C, three times daily. Then count the number of UTIs over six months without treatment. If you have fewer infections and no side effects, you may decide to continue use. I would start with mandelate and, if not effective, then try hippurate.

Take vitamin C alone: Vitamin C alone (500 to 1,000 mg twice a day) has been proposed to prevent UTIs by two mechanisms. First, it can be converted into ascorbic acid in the bladder, and if sufficient acidification occurs, it may prevent bacterial growth. Second, it's an antioxidant, which may restore the health of bladder tissue. There are, however, no strong studies showing a benefit of vitamin C alone; it is more effective when used with methenamine, as discussed above.

Take probiotics: Probiotics are cultures of bacteria thought to be beneficial by inhibiting bacteria that cause disease. In particular, certain strains of bacteria, such as *lactobacillus* (which is present in almost all yogurt), interfere with the colonization of the bladder by harmful bacteria such as *E. coli*. Studies using probiotics have yielded conflicting results, probably because the composition of probiotics is highly variable. The use of probiotics by mouth has shown no benefit. The best positive studies for probiotics have been in people who use vaginal suppositories containing live cultures at least twice weekly. You may consider performing your own test over six months to determine whether suppositories work for you.

Treatments That Are *Not* Recommended

Even with the best of intentions, many people will still have at least one UTI a year. Consequently, there are some preventive practices, *many of which I do not recommend*, that have become popular with both disabled and nondisabled people.

Antibiotics: Antibiotics should not be used as prevention but instead limited to situations in which a UTI is clearly present; there are simply too many harmful consequences of using antibiotics daily: 1) If you use the same antibiotic daily, it's likely that the bacteria will eventually become resistant to it; 2) Antibiotics modify the types of good bacteria present in your intestines (your gut microbiome), and changes in the gut microbiome can produce molecules that are harmful to other organs, such as the brain, heart, and liver. Antibiotics can also allow overgrowth of harmful bacteria such as *Clostridium difficile* (*C. diff*), which secretes a toxin that causes severe diarrhea and can lead to death; 3) Many antibiotics interfere with the metabolism of other drugs, which can cause toxic side effects. For example, the antibiotic ciprofloxacin (brand name Cipro) interacts with 129 different medications; and 4) Antibiotics can be expensive.

Cranberry: There are many studies of cranberry juice or concentrate, cranberry tablets, and cranberry capsules to prevent UTI. The studies included people with neurogenic bladder, women with recurrent UTIs, pregnant women, and cancer patients. In all groups, there was no benefit of taking cranberry for UTI prevention.

New Approaches on the Horizon

Three areas hold great promise for bladder health:

1. **Probiotics:** In addition to the bacteria present in the bladder, there are also bacteria present in your intestines, which are called the gut microbiome. It may become possible to identify the good and bad bacteria in your gut and use specific probiotics (or treatments that facilitate growth of beneficial bacteria) to increase the good bacteria and inhibit harmful bacterial growth in the bladder;

2. **Devices to control bladder function:** New devices may take advantage of the intact peripheral nerves and muscle in the bladder. In the future, we may implant biosensors, which can measure pressure and distension, in the bladder, and electrical stimulators that coordinate opening of the urethral sphincter and contraction of the bladder;

3. **Catheter material:** Materials used for catheters may be improved to make it more difficult for bacteria to adhere and may even slowly release medicines or compounds that prevent bacterial colonization and growth. Currently, many catheters are made with silver in them, but its efficacy is limited.

There's a powerful connection between your gastrointestinal system and your bladder, starting with periodontal health and ending with the bacteria in your colon. So it's not surprising that many people encounter similar problems with their gut—which will be explored in the next chapter.

———

Everything You Need to Know

For many, maintaining a healthy bladder can be a challenge. Since your bladder health is crucial to your overall health and longevity, as well as your quality of life, it's important to be vigilant in the areas that impact your bladder's function and susceptibility to infection.

If you're permanently incontinent, there are a number of options to consider, and it's important to be as informed as possible when you and your doctor discuss which ones you might try. There are advantages and disadvantages to virtually all of them, so your decision will depend on your personal priorities and what can work well for you in the long term.

Urinary tract infections are not an "inconvenience"—they are serious threats to your health. They can be difficult to diagnose accurately, so be sure you learn to recognize your own symptoms. Treatments vary as well; keep in mind that it's easy for a doctor to prescribe an antibiotic, but it's also far too easy for that approach to have negative consequences on your overall health. An ounce of prevention is worth a pound of cure.

As always, keep a notebook to record your health achievements and setbacks so that you can see what works best for you.

10

Digestive Tract Health

STILL REMEMBER CLEARLY how thrilled I was to be able to eat solid food after my injury. For six weeks, I had been receiving nourishment and calories from a feeding tube, and I dearly missed the pleasure of tasting, savoring, chewing, and swallowing food. My injury had made it impossible for me to swallow; I was told I would have to relearn how to do that—it wouldn't be automatic. The process would take time, but I was determined to enjoy meals with family and friends again. My first solid food? Chocolate pudding. I can still taste it!

Food is one of life's simple pleasures, a significant element of our quality of life, and the best way to nourish our bodies with the nutrients we need. Sure, there are supplements we can take, but none are as beneficial as real food itself. But after your injury swallowing can be difficult or even impossible, not only changing your entire relationship with food, but also affecting your digestive health.

Although many assume the digestive tract begins in the stomach, or even the small intestine, it actually begins in your mouth. After your injury, every part of the digestive tract—from your mouth to your rectum—may be dysfunctional. Chewing and swallowing, for example, might be difficult. While trouble swallowing limits what you can eat, it also poses a safety issue; not only can you choke on food, but it can also go into your lungs (aspiration), which can cause pneumonia (see Figure 14).

The anatomy of the gastrointestinal (GI) tract (Figure 21) is a series of connected tubes including the stomach, small intestine, colon, and rectum. The GI tract plays a key role in your absorption of nutrients and proper function of your immune system. The most common problem is constipation, which can be caused by a multitude of reasons: not moving or standing enough (and thus not allowing gravity to help move stool); weak core muscles; opiates and other drugs that slow stool movement; and dysfunction of the autonomic nervous system, which controls the muscle movement of the intestine and colon. Some people experience fecal incontinence, which is usually caused by loss of control of your anus, specifically the external sphincter muscle, which is controlled by the autonomic nervous system. Fecal incontinence and constipation are not inconveniences;

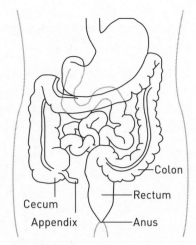

Figure 21. GI tract

they are potential health threats. You'll need to develop a "bowel program" so that you have regular bowel movements and avoid constipation or fecal incontinence.

Swallowing and Dysphagia

The psychological benefits of being able to eat and drink normally cannot be overstated. Even when you're in the hospital, the *pleasure* of eating is important. Eating is also a social opportunity that allows you to enjoy time with your friends and family. So, your health care team will be working to help you take food by mouth as soon as possible. Dysphagia, or difficulty in swallowing, is a common problem, and it can be described in three phases. In the first phase, food is placed in the mouth and kept there by the tongue and palate (oral cavity). This phase is voluntary and under our control. The second phase begins when food is transferred from the mouth into the throat (pharynx). The third phase occurs when the esophagus, a muscular tube that produces waves of coordinated contractions, pushes the food down. As the esophagus contracts, a muscular valve at the end opens and allows the food to enter the stomach.

Oropharyngeal dysphagia is characterized by difficulty initiating a swallow, which is the most common problem. Swallowing may be accompanied by coughing, choking, aspiration, and a sensation of food remaining in the throat. Many people, myself included, have these problems, especially with liquids, chewy foods like white bread and apple skin, and large pills. Chewable pills were developed to help people with dysphagia.

Esophageal dysphagia, characterized by difficulty swallowing, causes the feeling that food is stuck in your throat several seconds after you start to swallow. This is a painful problem that most people deal with by trying to cough up and spit out the pill or food.

Aspiration: Dysphagia isn't only unpleasant; it can actually be harmful when it leads to aspiration, which is when something enters your airway or lungs by accident. During the process of swallowing, the epiglottis (a valve over the windpipe, or trachea) must come down and direct the food into the esophagus and stomach. If this doesn't occur, due to dysphagia, the food will go into your lungs instead. It's also possible that the contents of your stomach can be regurgitated into your esophagus and then down into your lungs. These scenarios can lead to a serious medical complication: aspiration pneumonia. This is particularly harmful, since the lungs become stiffer (harder to inflate) after pneumonia. If you have underlying respiratory problems—either control of breathing by the brain or diaphragm dysfunction due to nerve injury—this makes the lifetime risk of pneumonia much greater (more on this on page 167).

Prevalence: If you're experiencing dysphagia, you face potentially life-threatening complications. There are two significant predictors of risk for dysphagia: age and tracheostomy with mechanical ventilation. Additional risk factors include spinal surgery via an anterior cervical approach for SCI (likely in tetraplegics with injuries to the neck), and low scores on cognitive ability and level of consciousness (Glasgow coma scale) for TBI and stroke. Many stroke and TBI patients also have difficulties with swallowing because the action is complex; damage in many parts of the brain (brain stem, thalamus, basal ganglia, limbic system, cerebellum, and motor and sensory cortices) can cause problems in different phases of swallowing. In particular, patients who have a tracheostomy and low cognitive function are at the highest risk.

If you have depressed coughing reflexes, the aspiration of food and stomach acid may occur silently, which is why you should have a swallowing study performed in the hospital prior to starting to eat food again. The best test is a video fluoroscopic swallowing study, a relatively simple test in which a thick mixture containing barium is swallowed and the motion of the barium down the throat and esophagus is followed by using a video X-ray. The time to initiate a swallow, transfer into the stomach, and the size of the bolus (the amount of mixture) are key measures of difficulty swallowing.

Management and treatment: Because of the severity of my injury, my team waited about two weeks to begin my swallowing exercises. The good news is that these exercises, usually taught by a speech pathologist, can both strengthen normal swallowing *and* teach you compensatory ways to swallow. The exact exercises and maneuvers that work are specific to each individual, and they progress from strengthening the muscles all the way to learning new ways of swallowing that prevent aspiration. Traditional dysphagia rehab therapies include chin tuck, effortful swallow, head tilt, head turn, supraglottic swallow, and the Mendelsohn and Masako (tongue hold) maneuvers. In my situation, the Masako maneuver—in which I held my tongue between my teeth while swallowing—was hugely helpful. I also learned effortful swallow, in which I had to squeeze my throat muscles as hard as I could while swallowing, because food would get stuck in the back of my throat. All these years later, I'm still careful to chew my food well, swallow carefully, and not talk while eating. Certain foods are particularly high-risk for me, including soft bread and spaghetti, both of which can get stuck in my throat.

The Neurogenic Bowel

Restoring bowel function has an enormous impact on your quality of life. Normal bowel function requires the brain and peripheral nervous system (together called the autonomic nervous system; Figure 6) to work properly, so those who have experienced an ANI are at risk for impaired bowel function. Most people suffer from constipation, though some will experience fecal incontinence. The two represent the ends of the normal spectrum, but fecal incontinence can be particularly challenging in terms of a normal social life. It's important to note that constipation is common in the general population and increases with age, as you get older, constipation may become *more* of a problem. But it can almost always be treated with nonpharmacologic interventions (see page 148). In contrast, fecal incontinence is more complex and requires greater adherence to strict therapeutic interventions (see page 152).

Assessing the neurogenic bowel: Assessment of your bowel function should be done by your primary care physician annually or when a significant change in your function occurs. While you may consider examinations of your anus and questions regarding your bowel movements embarrassing, it's critical that you have a thorough examination every year. As we grow older, gastrointestinal problems increase steadily; such that by age sixty-five, half of the general population has a history of gastrointestinal problems and nearly a third are actively being treated for a problem.

At least three examinations of bowel function should be performed yearly: a rectal exam including anal sphincter tone; a stool test for blood beginning at age fifty; and a colonoscopy every five years beginning at age fifty (or earlier, if you have a family history of colon cancer or severe constipation). The need for colonoscopy should be weighed with the difficulties associated with this test, because the bowel preparation and anesthesia may be too exhausting and risky; your doctor will discuss the pros and cons with you.

Developing and evaluating an effective bowel program: For effective management of your bowel function, you'll need a bowel program. A successful bowel program should provide predictable and reliable results, take less than thirty minutes per day, have minimal side effects, and require the fewest number of medications and surgeries. To design an effective bowel program, consider your functional abilities, including your ability to sit (your balance and endurance), your arm and hand strength and dexterity, your ability to transfer if you're in a wheelchair, and the condition of your skin. You should also consider your diet, frequency of bowel movements, consistency of stool, ability to exercise and stand, and any medications you may be taking. Because bowel function is so heavily influenced by these factors, changes in bowel function can occur frequently, and when that happens, you'll need to revisit your plan.

Constipation: Many factors cause constipation, with age at the top of the list. If you have any *two* of the following—straining, hard stools, sensation of incomplete evacuation, sensation of a blockage in the rectum, and fewer than three bowel movements per week—you are experiencing constipation. Without even thinking about it, healthy people use several maneuvers to help achieve normal bowel movements: They sit up and lean forward on the toilet seat, squeeze their stomach muscles, and take a deep breath before squeezing (a Valsalva maneuver). But after your injury, you may not have the strength or coordination to do these things. If this is the case, part of your PT program should be to regain these functions or develop compensatory approaches. For example, digital stimulation of the anus and rectum (inserting a finger into the anus and gently pushing against the rectum several times), abdominal pressure, and caffeinated coffee or tea can help initiate a bowel movement. Suppositories and enemas may be useful to start a bowel movement and soften the stool (see page 151).

Diet and nutrition: What you eat plays a major role in the composition of stool as well as its movement through your intestines. But the same diet can result in differences in bowel movement among any two individuals, so any diet will likely need to be modified for you. Work with a registered dietitian to develop a diet that helps your bowel program. Let's start with fiber. Most dietary fiber isn't digested or absorbed; it's combined with other products of digested food and bacteria to form stool and regulate its consistency. For nondisabled people, fiber intake of 20 to 25 grams per day is recommended. There are two types of fiber: soluble, which is found in fruits, oats, barley, peas, and beans; and insoluble, which is found in many whole grains, such as wheat, rye, rice, and oats, as well as flaxseeds. Soluble fiber dissolves in water to make a gel that may reduce blood cholesterol and sugar, thereby maintaining lower blood glucose and preventing diabetes. Insoluble fiber attracts water into your colon, making your stool softer and preventing constipation.

In general, fruits and vegetables are very useful in preventing constipation. To determine the correct amount of fiber in your diet, keep a weekly food diary. Generally, recommendations include starting with at least 15 grams of fiber per day, then increasing it by 5 grams every two weeks (and consuming at least 25 grams daily as a goal); keep a journal to monitor stool consistency and side effects on a daily basis. Be aware that increased fiber intake can lead to side effects, like bloating and flatulence. Cramping pain can occur with certain types of fiber, such as flax. But these should disappear as your body adapts and your bowel health improves.

Two other important considerations in your diet are your consumption of animal products and your fluid intake. In general, meat (beef, pork, lamb, chicken) is more constipating than seafood. Meat also alters the composition of the bacteria in your intestine, which affects the formation and consistency of stool. (Refer back to chapters 6 and 8 for more on healthy diets, like the Mediterranean, DASH, and Chinese diets.) To keep your stools soft, which makes moving your bowels easier, it's essential that you consume enough fluids (eight 8-ounce servings of water) each day. This may be a problem if you're restricting fluids to decrease urine output when performing self-catheterization. The amount of fluid you need depends on your health, how active you are, and your local climate. This is a subject to discuss with your health care team.

Developing a bowel program for constipation: While your injury may have altered your normal daily routine, it is important to establish a regular schedule for your bowel program, and it should allow for a *minimum* of three bowel movements each week. (My program allows for bowel movements on Tuesday, Thursday, and Saturday, so that during the work week I have only two "long" mornings in the bathroom.)

It's essential that you do your bowel movement program at the same time, whether it's every day or every other day. The optimal time for your bowel movements is within the first two hours after you wake up (and after you've eaten breakfast) because the colon is most active first thing in the morning and after a meal. During the work week, I'm usually in a rush to get to my office, so on Tuesdays and Thursdays I speed things up by using a Magic Bullet suppository and drinking a cup of coffee as soon as I wake up.

Exercise and standing: You can greatly improve your intestinal motility with exercise and standing, which can be incorporated into your bowel program. There are many kinds of exercise that stimulate the bowels; the best ones are those that increase your heart rate and cause you to use your breathing muscles, and even better, your abdominal muscles. These exercises activate receptors that cause the muscles that line your intestine to contract, and they strengthen the muscles necessary to help squeeze your abdomen and your lower diaphragm, which creates pressure that helps propel the stools down and out.

Standing is perhaps the simplest way to improve bowel function. Without any other effort on your part, gravity helps your stool move through your intestines. Even if you're unable to move your legs, you may be able to use a standing frame, with assistance (ask your physical therapist). I use a standing frame to stand for one hour each day (Figure 22). The top serves as a desk so that I can work while standing. It only takes two minutes to get on and off, using a transfer board.

In addition to improving bowel function, standing prevents bone

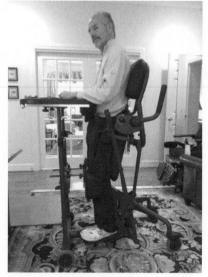

Figure 22. Standing frame

loss (osteoporosis), because it's a weight-bearing exercise; it improves heart and lung function; and it just feels good. But be aware that your blood pressure must be carefully monitored while you're standing to avoid fainting. Time of day is important too—standing after a big meal is *not* a good idea. Avoid standing during hot weather, after taking medications that lower your blood pressure, or when you're dehydrated.

Medications: In most cases, medications should be a last resort for improving bowel function. That said, there are several that can be useful for a practical and effective bowel program. They are listed here in the order that they should be tried, based on their efficacy and safety.

A typical American diet (low in fiber, high in meat) produces harder stools, which makes them more difficult to move and increases your risk of hemorrhoids. The two most common drugs to help soften stool are docusate sodium (Colace) and docusate calcium (Surfak); they work by decreasing reabsorption of water in the colon, thereby softening the stool. Increasing the absorption of water increases the stool volume, causing the walls of the intestine to expand and stimulating movement of the stool. The most common over-the-counter products to help in this regard are psyllium (Metamucil; Perdiem) and methylcellulose (Citrucel). Be sure to drink extra fluids when using these supplements.

You can also use laxatives to stimulate bowel motility. Personally, I prefer laxatives that contain polyethylene glycol (MiraLax, Glycolax), which do not cause gas or bloating. Faster-acting are the saline laxatives, which include magnesium hydroxide (Milk of Magnesia) and magnesium citrate. Magnesium citrate can cause a bowel movement in as quickly as one hour after drinking it. Stimulant laxatives promote stool movement by irritating the bowel; these include senna—Ex-Lax, Fletcher's Laxative (formerly Castoria), Senokot—and bisacodyl (Correctol, Dulcolax). It's important to use these the day *before* your bowel program only, because excessive use can decrease bowel motility and dilate the bowel.

Some people use suppositories or enemas for bowel movements. (Personally, I find enemas messy and not as effective as pills or suppositories.) The best known enema is saline solution (Fleet). The most common suppository is bisacodyl, which comes with either a vegetable oil base (Dulcolax) or a polyethylene glycol base (Magic Bullet). I like the Magic Bullet due to its rapid onset of action, which is usually less than thirty minutes. I don't recommend using mineral oil to soften stools, as it's less reliable and can be potentially harmful.

Fecal Incontinence

Diagnosis: Fecal incontinence is the loss of voluntary control over bowel movements. The most common cause of fecal incontinence is a loss of control of your anal sphincter. This is most prevalent in people with complete SCI. However, it may also be due to diseases of the intestines, such as gluten and lactose intolerance. Finally, it may be due to other foods in your diet that stimulate contractions of your intestine, such as coffee and tea. To determine the cause, your doctor will examine your colon. This is usually performed using colonoscopy, which not only shows your doctor the entire colon, but also allows for biopsy, if needed, to determine if there's an underlying illness. Other imaging techniques include ultrasound, CT scan, and magnetic resonance imaging (MRI). Anorectal manometry measures the pressure in different parts of the colon to identify the anatomic site of the problem. It's especially useful to assess the tone of the anal sphincters, which can also be used to determine if rectal sensation and rectal reflexes are impaired.

Make it easy to find the toilet: One of the easiest solutions for fecal incontinence is to use a bedside commode, especially if you have limited mobility. Many people will experience a delayed sense of when they need to go; by the time they feel the urge to defecate, stool may already be in the rectum. If you're in bed, the time it takes to get out of bed, find a walker or your wheelchair, and get to the bathroom may be so long that you aren't able to maintain enough anal sphincter control to prevent an accident.

Diet: The foods you eat play a critical role in fecal incontinence, but just like constipation, your diet must be individualized working with a registered dietitian. Start by determining whether you're lactose or gluten intolerant, as these intolerances can cause abdominal cramping and diarrhea in many people. Spicy foods, fatty foods, caffeine, and alcohol can also increase stool frequency. Large meals stimulate the bowel, so eating several smaller meals throughout the day can be helpful.

Medical therapy: The three medical approaches to fecal incontinence are to increase stool volume, decrease frequency, and slow down bowel motility. The most common substances to increase stool volume are psyllium (Metamucil, Perdiem) and methylcellulose (Citrucel). Drugs for diarrhea, such as loperamide (Imodium) and diphenoxylate-atropine (Lomotil), can also decrease stool frequency, although they can also cause drowsiness. You can take an anticholinergic drug like hyoscyamine, which slows motility, prior to eating a meal.

Biofeedback: Biofeedback is a safe and noninvasive way that can help you identify and contract the anal sphincter muscles, which helps maintain continence. During biofeedback training, a pressure sensor is placed in the anus, where it can detect changes in pressure as you try to squeeze your anal sphincter muscles. You measure your progress using a pressure recording chart as you squeeze for thirty to sixty seconds to strengthen the muscles.

Surgery: The most invasive and helpful surgery is the colostomy, which requires general anesthesia. During the procedure, a part of the distal colon is attached to the abdominal wall, where stool collects in an external bag that is tightly attached to the skin. A good friend of mine had this done because he had a pressure ulcer that wouldn't heal due to fecal incontinence. Most people would have had the colostomy reversed once the pressure ulcer healed, but he found that it was so beneficial for his mental health that he kept it! The drawbacks, however, include the need to change the bag three to four times daily, a frequent odor, and, perhaps, unpleasant body image as a result. Each person's bowel program will differ; for him and many others, the convenience of the bag and lack of fecal incontinence outweigh the problems.

Bowel Management Outside the Home

The simplest approach to bowel management when you're away from home is to have established an effective bowel program. I know approximately how much stool I should eliminate each time I perform my bowel program. If I don't have adequate elimination, I remain on the toilet for up to fifteen minutes longer than my usual thirty minutes. If I still haven't gone, I wear disposable absorbent briefs (Depend, for example), just in case I have some leakage.

When I travel, I have a bowel movement on the morning I depart, so that I don't have to have another one until two or even three mornings later. If I'll be away for longer than that, I have a lightweight travel chair that fits in a rolling suitcase and fits over most toilets (it also serves as a shower chair). It's common to become dehydrated while traveling, especially on long plane flights, so I try to drink extra fluids (at least 16 ounces more than usual). You can also increase the amount of bowel stimulants (senna) and stool bulk formers (Miralax) if you're unable to maintain a good bowel program while traveling.

It's a Journey

After six weeks in the hospital, when I finally began to eat, I had a bowel movement every night after dinner and had to sleep wearing a diaper. Remarkably, within a few weeks of eating solid foods, I began to have regular bowel movements (every morning after breakfast), thanks to a regimen of stool softeners and bowel stimulants and a high-fiber diet. At first, I used a bedpan, then a bedside commode when I regained the ability to sit up. I eventually transitioned to using a shower chair as a seat over a regular toilet. Although I learned to surrender my modesty and my initial despair over what I felt was a loss of personal dignity, I continue to work on a plan for an independent bowel program. I'm almost there but can't yet achieve complete elimination by myself. I think I still need stronger abdominal muscles.

For many years now, a routine bowel program that I manage myself has been part of my routine; sleeping in a diaper seems like something from a lifetime ago. Remember: Recovery is all about accepting the formerly unacceptable as you navigate this journey.

Everything You Need to Know

Good digestive-tract health is essential to your overall health. What you eat affects every aspect of your recovery.

- After your injury, your swallowing may be impaired (dysphagia). There is effective treatment, but first the underlying physiologic deficits must be identified during a formal swallowing evaluation.

- Traditional therapies focus on prevention of secondary complications such as aspiration and pneumonia, with the long-term aim of improved swallowing and control.

- Constipation is a common condition and poses real health threats if not addressed. An episodic approach won't help you in the long term; develop and follow a bowel program that works for your lifestyle. Your health care team can help you create a plan that allows you to have regular, predictable bowel movements. This achievement will not only support better overall health but also improve your quality of life.

- Fecal incontinence can occur after your injury. There are a number of approaches to address it. Discuss your options with your health care team to find out which options appeal to you.

11

Heart Health

D ID YOU KNOW THAT your injury significantly increases your risk of heart attack and stroke compared to your nondisabled contemporaries? The reasons are unknown, but the possibilities include chronic inflammation (frequently associated with obesity), autonomic dysfunction (especially blood pressure oscillations), and the fact that the greatest risk for a heart attack or stroke is having a history of either one.

Aggressive prevention (and treatment, if needed) of heart disease and its risk factors should now be part of your daily routine. The risk factors for heart attack or stroke are the same for you as they are for the rest of the population—smoking, high total cholesterol, high blood pressure, a family history of heart attack and stroke, and poorly controlled type 2 diabetes—but they now present an even *greater* danger to you. So, if any one of these descriptions applies to you, it's time to address them.

In addition to quitting smoking (if you smoke), eating a healthy diet and getting regular exercise are at the top of the prevention list. If it is determined that you should be taking medicine to lessen your risk factors, your doctor will discuss the risks of these drugs with you, since the side effects can be greater after ANI. For example, hypertension is a major risk factor for heart attack and stroke. However, in the presence of autonomic dysfunction, your blood pressure can rapidly go down. The autonomic nervous system regulates your heart rate, which should increase when your blood pressure goes down, but may fail to do so after your injury.

The Cardiovascular System

Anatomy: The cardiovascular system (Figure 23) refers to the heart, blood vessels, and blood; it includes the major vessels that supply the abdomen, legs, arms, brain, and heart. In SCI, bleeding into the spinal cord compresses the nerves and deprives them of oxygen; in stroke, clotting of a blood vessel due to atherosclerosis (fat buildup and inflammation in the artery wall) or bleeding through a hole in the artery wall (hemorrhage) deprives nerves of oxygen and releases toxic substances that kill nerves; and in TBI, both bleeding *and* clotting contribute to nerve damage and nerve death. Though not explicitly part of the cardiovascular system, the kidneys are crucial for cardiovascular health; kidney dysfunction causes hypertension, which damages vessels, making them susceptible to atherosclerosis, which contributes to heart attack and stroke.

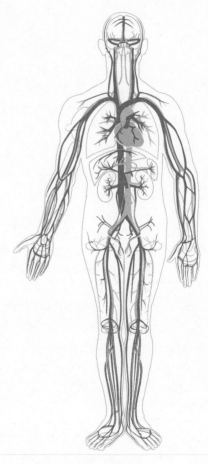

Figure 23. Cardiovascular system

Heart Problems

Cardiovascular disease (CVD) is the leading cause of death in the US, and it's also responsible for the greatest number of deaths in those who have experienced an ANI. CVD includes stroke, aneurysm, coronary artery disease (CAD), heart attack, peripheral vascular disease, heart failure, and arrhythmias. Traditional risk factors cause even *more* harm in people with ANI.

Relative Risk of CVD in ANI

The relative risk of CVD varies widely depending on whether you've had an SCI, TBI, or stroke. If you've had a stroke, you're at increased risk for a second stroke. If you've had a SCI, the increase in CVD is largely related to heart attacks caused by atherosclerosis in the coronary arteries (CAD). As a cardiologist, I believe that the primary reason for increased CAD is autonomic dysfunction. If you've had a stroke, the cause in 85 percent of people is an ischemic stroke, which is due to atherosclerosis in the arteries of the brain. The larger vessels, such as the carotid and the middle cerebral arteries, are most susceptible to atherosclerosis. This is especially unfortunate because blood flow from these vessels provides nutrients and oxygen to almost 25 percent of your brain. If you've had a TBI, there are few long-term risks of CVD, except if you have autonomic dysfunction.

It's important to understand that you can achieve a *dramatic* reduction in your risk of death from CVD or CAD by modifying your lifestyle. If anything in the following list (ranked from highest to lowest risk) has your name on it, it's time to make some changes:

- type 2 diabetes, both insulin–requiring and treatable with drugs
- smoking
- high total cholestrol
- hypertension
- overweight and obesity
- unhealthy diet
- physical inactivity

Type 2 diabetes: If you have type 2 diabetes, your body either resists the effects of insulin, which regulates the movement of sugar into your cells, or doesn't produce enough insulin to maintain normal glucose levels. It's commonly associated with obesity. Diabetes increases the risk of CAD and heart attack by three to four times. High levels of circulating glucose damage blood vessels throughout the body, accelerating the process of atherosclerosis in the heart, brain, and kidneys. Exercise can help avoid this, because it stimulates uptake of glucose by your muscles, but you may not be able to exercise very well after your injury. Plus, the majority of skeletal muscle mass is found in the legs, and both SCI and stroke frequently cause atrophy of the leg muscles.

Treating type 2 diabetes is more difficult if you've suffered an ANI. While there are many effective medications for lowering glucose that have beneficial effects (decreasing heart failure and CVD events), others have harmful side effects (increasing fluid in your legs, low blood sugar, skin rash or itching, sensitivity to sunlight, upset stomach, and weight gain). Therefore, the choice of medication needs to be individualized, something your primary care physician and a diabetes specialist (an endocrinologist) can determine.

Smoking: Smoking is one of the major risk factors for CVD, and the risk is strongly related to the number of cigarettes you smoke each day and number of years you've been smoking. Cigarette smoke causes inflammation in the blood vessels and directly activates inflammatory white blood cells, leading to CVD. The treatment is simple: Stop smoking! I know, that's easier said than done. Smoking is addictive, so stopping can be difficult. But it's worth the effort; the benefits are rapid, and within five years of quitting smoking, a study showed that participants had a 13 percent reduction in the risk of death from all causes, a 27 percent reduction from stroke, and a 47 percent reduction from heart disease–related deaths.[1]

To quit smoking, set a quit date and talk to your doctor in advance. A two-pronged approach is best: 1) Change habits that trigger your desire for a cigarette, and 2) Try a smoking-cessation medicine. If you always have a cigarette after lunch, for example, take a five-minute walk instead. Ask your doctor for a medication that will help diminish the craving for cigarettes and the symptoms of withdrawal, such as anxiety. Many doctors use Wellbutrin (bupropion) and Chantix (varenicline), because they appear to be more effective than over-the-counter therapies such as nicotine patches and gum. Start these medications at least two weeks before your quit date; otherwise, the withdrawal symptoms that are greatest in the first three days are more likely to cause you to give up. It's so much harder to quit if someone in your household smokes, so make it a family affair and vow to quit together. Support each other through the transition to becoming nonsmokers.

High cholestrol: Total cholesterol should be the initial blood test because it does not require you to fast. Cholesterol is an essential building block for all of our cells. Your liver makes proteins called lipoproteins that carry cholesterol to your cells for their use. When we talk about our cholesterol levels, we're referring to two important lipoproteins: 1) low-density lipoprotein (LDL, the "bad" one), and 2) high-density lipoprotein (HDL, the "good" one). We measure blood cholesterol because of the direct relationship between the level of LDL and the presence of CVD. If you can't bring high LDL levels down to the normal range by making changes to your diet and lifestyle, your doctor will prescribe medication to help.

Hypertension: Hypertension, or high blood pressure, is a major risk factor for CAD and stroke, which is why it's important for you to pay attention to your numbers. Treat if they are greater than 130/90. The first actions in treating hypertension are lifestyle modifications: consuming a low-salt diet, regular exercise, weight loss, decreasing stress and improving your coping skills, and getting plenty of sleep. If these methods aren't successful in reducing your blood pressure, your doctor may start anti-hypertensive drug therapy.

Overweight and obesity: The best way to determine if you are at an unhealthy weight is by assessing central obesity, which looks at the body's distribution of fat. Increased central obesity is indicated by a waist circumference greater than 40 inches (100 cm) in men and greater than 35 inches (90 cm) in women. Carrying more fat around the waist increases your CVD risk. Treating obesity and maintaining weight loss is difficult, but exercise and a healthy diet are the best routes to take. If you are capable of regular exercise, moderate to vigorous intensity physical exercise for at least forty minutes most days of the week is recommended. A Mediterranean diet (see page 95) that emphasizes vegetables, fruits, legumes, and whole grains is an excellent way to maintain an optimal weight.

Physical inactivity: Exercise is key to a healthy lifestyle for anyone, and that's particularly true after your injury. Make it part of your weekly routine. Workouts of thirty to sixty minutes per session, three to seven times a week, are essential for your heart health. Your exercises can include hand-crank ergometry, hand cycling, swimming, and functional electrical stimulation of muscles. If you have incomplete neurologic deficits, like me, you may be able to do more intense exercise, such as cycling using a recumbent tricycle; walking with a cane, crutches, or walker; adaptive sit-skiing; kayaking; and rowing. Body weight–supported walking overground or treadmill training is excellent, but it requires the assistance of one or more therapists.

Orthostatic hypotension: This problem is a decrease in systolic blood pressure (the first number of the two that measure your blood pressure) of more than 20 or a decrease in diastolic blood pressure (the second number) of more than 10 when going from lying down to sitting up. Typical symptoms are fatigue, weakness, dizziness, light-headedness, and blurred vision. When I stand up and my blood pressure drops, I experience blurred vision and need to sit down quickly. There have been several occasions when I've fainted and fallen, due to autonomic dysfunction.

It's normal for your blood pressure to decrease when you stand up, because blood accumulates in the legs. Your autonomic nervous system (ANS) senses the drop and activates the sympathetic nervous system to increase heart rate, stimulate contraction of the heart, and decrease blood flow to the gut and skin. But after your injury, your body may not be able to sense the drop or activate the ANS. The good news is there are many simple treatments, including compression stockings on the legs, an abdominal binder, adequate fluid intake, avoiding alcohol and caffeine, and increased salt intake. Rarely, drugs, such as alpha adrenergic agonists (midodrine), or mineralocorticoid agents (fludrocortisone), are needed to address the problem—you can discuss this with your doctor.

Diagnosis and Evaluation of Heart Disease

People with ANI often have unusual symptoms or no symptoms of coronary artery disease (CAD) at all. Therefore, the best tests don't depend on symptoms—but they can be seen with imaging. CAD testing frequently involves a stress to increase heart rate, typically walking on a treadmill. But if you're unable to walk, the stress will have to be induced by arm exercise or by using a drug to speed up the heart.

Echocardiogram: An echocardiogram is an ultrasound measurement of the heart. It's a noninvasive test that indicates the contractility of the heart, the structure of its upper and lower chambers, and the heart valves. The velocity of blood flow can be measured using the Doppler technique, which shows whether the heart valves are normal, leaking, or narrowed. This information is important, because CAD can be diagnosed if regions of the heart show diminished contraction.

Exercise tolerance test (ETT): Making the heart work harder increases the likelihood of detecting CAD, so ETT is the usual approach. If you are physically able, you'll wear electrocardiogram (ECG or EKG) electrodes and start to walk on a treadmill at a slow pace. Every three minutes, the pace is increased until you become tired or have symptoms like chest pain, left arm pain, or shortness of breath. If CAD is present, the ECG will show specific changes. The ETT can be combined with echocardiography or with injection of a nuclear medicine to provide images of the regions most affected by CAD. These tests are also routine after stroke.

Computerized tomography (CT) calcium score: A cardiac CT scan for coronary calcium is a noninvasive way of obtaining information about the presence, location, and extent of calcified atherosclerosis in the coronary arteries. Because calcium is a marker of CAD, the amount of calcium detected on a cardiac CT scan is a helpful prognostic tool. The more coronary calcium you have, the more likely you will have CAD problems in the future.

Cardiac catheterization and angiogram: To locate the exact places in your coronary arteries where the atherosclerosis has increased so much that it narrows the artery, your doctor will perform imaging of the coronary arteries. A catheter is inserted into the openings of the three coronary arteries, and X-ray contrast dye is injected to show where there is significant narrowing (a 70 percent or greater decrease in the diameter of the artery).

ANI-Specific Heart Health Problems

SCI

Autonomic dysreflexia (AD): If your SCI is above T6, you may experience AD, which is characterized by increased blood pressure (20 to 40 mm Hg above baseline), severe headache, and loss of skin color below the level of injury with flushing and sweating above the level of lesion. The major risk of AD is extreme elevations of blood pressure (250 to 300 mm Hg systolic, and 200 to 220 mm Hg diastolic). AD can cause seizures and bleeding in the brain from a ruptured blood vessel. As a result, everyone with SCI should carry an automated blood pressure cuff (Omron is a good brand), to check their blood pressure when they experience AD symptoms. AD is usually provoked by dysfunction of an internal organ, leading to severe activation of the ANS. Common causes include bladder distention, fecal impaction, and pressure sores (more on this in chapter 13). Treatment of AD should be focused on identifying and fixing the cause simultaneously, and on lowering the blood pressure. If the problem is bladder distention, a Foley catheter should be inserted to drain the bladder; if the cause is fecal impaction, an enema should be administered immediately. There are many ways to lower blood pressure, but intravenous injection is mandatory, in my opinion. At my hospital, we commonly use intravenous labetalol.

Bradycardia: Bradycardia is a slower-than-normal heartbeat. If you have an SCI, you are more susceptible to bradycardia. This is usually asymptomatic. If you rapidly change position from lying down to standing up, the usual response is for your heart rate to increase to maintain your blood pressure. With bradycardia, if your heart rate doesn't go up, you'll feel dizzy and might even faint.

No nighttime decrease in blood pressure: In most healthy people, blood pressure drops during sleep. But this decrease may not occur if your ANS is impaired, especially if you have a cervical SCI. Because this loss of the nighttime dip is associated with more CVD events, you should measure your blood pressure continuously for one to two days with an ambulatory blood pressure monitor if you have symptoms of autonomic dysfunction.

Temperature regulation: It's the job of the ANS to regulate and maintain a body temperature of 98.6°F (37°C), especially when the air temperature increases or when you become hot due to exertion. The two primary ways the ANS cools down the body are by diverting blood flow to the skin and increasing sweating. But both of these responses are impaired after SCI above T6 due to autonomic dysfunction. Failure to maintain normal body temperature can result in heat stroke, which is a body temperature greater than 104°F (40°C) and mental confusion. If not treated promptly, heat stroke can rapidly lead to severe organ damage and death. If you suspect you have heat stroke, seek emergency treatment; doctors will administer intravenous infusion of cold saline and place you in an ice water bath.

Stroke

Atrial fibrillation (AF): AF is the most common cause of an abnormal heartbeat (arrhythmia) in adults, and it significantly increases the risk of stroke. AF refers to the loss of the normal electrical and contractile properties of the atrium (the upper chamber of the heart). It has several causes, including hypertension, congestive heart failure, valvular heart disease, and heart attack. As a result, the normal contraction of the atrium is lost, so blood can clot, especially in the atrial appendage, a small pouch at the top of the atrium. These clots can dislodge and travel from the heart to the carotid arteries, then onward to the brain, where they cause a stroke,

Risk of AF and Treatment Guidelines

To predict the risk of stroke in patients with AF, doctors use the CHA2DS2-VASc score (Table 2). Current guidelines recommend that if the patient has a CHA2DS2-VASc score of 2 and above, oral anticoagulation therapy should be started. Typical drugs would be a vitamin K antagonist (e.g., warfarin) or a direct oral anticoagulant drug (e.g., dabigatran, rivaroxaban, edoxaban, or apixaban). The choice of drug is complex and requires an honest discussion with your cardiologist.

by blocking either a major artery or multiple smaller arteries. The best treatment for AF is individualized, based on the underlying cause, coexisting medical conditions, frequency of AF, and patient preferences. Therefore, consultation with a cardiologist is necessary if you are diagnosed with this condition.

	Condition	Points
C	Congestive heart failure (or left ventricular systolic dysfunction)	1
H	Hypertension: blood pressure consistently above 140/90 mmHg (or treated hypertension on medication	1
A_2	Age ≥ 75	2
D	Diabetes Mellitus	1
S_2	Prior stroke or TIA or thromboembolism	2
V	Vascular disease (e.g., peripheral artery disease, myocardial infarction, aortic plaque)	1
A	Age 65–74 years	1
Sc	Sex category (i.e., female sex)	1

Table 2: Risk predictor for thromboembolic stroke; CHA2DS2-VASc score

Traumatic Brain Injury

Systemic inflammatory response syndrome (SIRS): SIRS is a severe systemic disease that frequently progresses to sepsis. Sepsis is caused by infections such as severe pneumonia or UTI, while SIRS can be caused by infections or severe trauma. A SIRS diagnosis requires two or more of the following: 1) heart rate greater than 90 beats per minute, 2) respiratory rate greater than 20 breaths per minute, 3) temperature less than 96.8°F (36°C) or greater than 100.4°F (38°C), and 4) white blood cell count less than 4,000 cells/mm^3 or greater than 12,000 cells/mm^3). Early SIRS is common in people with moderate to severe TBI, and the presence of SIRS is associated with decreased heart function that may lead to multi-organ failure, especially of the kidney and lungs. The good news is that SIRS usually resolves on its own within one week, but it's an important condition to be aware of and to discuss with your doctor.

———

Everything You Need to Know

After SCI or stroke, you have a significantly increased risk of heart attack or stroke. As a result, you'll need to make lifestyle changes, such as consuming a healthier diet; getting regular exercise; treating medical problems like hypertension, diabetes, and elevated cholesterol; and if you smoke, quitting.

Traumatic brain injury doesn't increase your risk of cardiovascular disease, but if prior to or after your injury you had or have any of the risk factors listed below, you are at an increased risk of heart attack or stroke:

- type 2 diabetes
- smoking
- high LDL cholesterol
- a family history of cardiovascular disease
- excess weight or obesity
- lack of regular exercise
- an unhealthy diet
- atrial fibrillation (for stroke only)

Also, many people with ANI have autonomic nervous system (ANS) dysfunction. This manifests most commonly by orthostatic hypotension and fluctuations in blood pressure. After SCI, ANS dysfunction may become life threatening due to autonomic dysreflexia, in which your systolic blood pressure can rise as high as 300 mm Hg, necessitating emergency treatment.

The good news for all of us is that our heart health is primarily determined by our lifestyle and the choices we make on a daily basis. This means you can decrease your risk of heart attack or stroke by modifying your habits. Be sure to reach out for help in any of the areas where you know you need to make changes; your family, friends, and health care team will support you.

12

Lung Health

As we breathe, our lungs exchange carbon dioxide that our tissues produce for oxygen, which the body uses to metabolize food for energy. The lungs themselves are not affected by ANI, but the *muscles* that help them do their work—the diaphragm and other muscles in the chest and abdomen—can be paralyzed, causing lung dysfunction. The two major problems that you may experience are mechanical: the physical movement of air in and out of your body and the risk of pneumonia. There have been remarkable improvements in preventing hospital-acquired pneumonia, which dramatically reduces the long-term problems caused by mechanical ventilation and infection.

Lung Problems

Mechanical problems: In people with SCI and TBI, the trauma from the event that caused the injury may break the ribs. This can puncture the lungs and cause bleeding into the chest that "squeezes" air out of the lungs, resulting in their collapse. If enough ribs are broken, the integrity of the chest wall will be destroyed so that it can no longer cohesively move in and out, causing a mechanical failure of lung ventilation. Treatment consists of a three eighths–inch tube inserted between the ribs and into the space between the chest wall and the collapsed lung to drain the blood and other fluids. The tube is connected to suction to speed up the drainage, which will require two to three days. A chest X-ray will monitor re-expansion of the lung, at which point the tube can be removed.

Hospital-acquired pneumonia is a lung infection acquired in the hospital more than forty-eight hours after admission. This type of pneumonia is usually more severe than other types for two reasons. First, you are already in the hospital for an illness that causes significant stress to your body's immune system. Second, the organisms that cause infections in the hospital may be more resistant to antibiotics. After ANI, you're especially prone to pneumonia because of five breathing problems:

- mechanical ventilation (being on a ventilator)
- secretions (fluid from the lungs that can clog the breathing tubes)
- atelectasis (collapse of parts of the lung)
- aspiration (food and material from your stomach and mouth get into your lungs; Figure 14)
- obstructive sleep apnea (periods when breathing stops while sleeping, which predisposes you to heart and lung problems; see page 000)

Treatment is similar for patients on and off ventilators. Because the incidence of multi-drug-resistant bacteria is very high, the choice of antibiotics must be individualized based on the type of bacteria that are found in sputum and blood cultures, combined with knowledge of which antibiotics the bacteria are resistant to. Usually, treatment lasts for seven days. Recovery is best assessed by patient symptoms (temperature, heart rate, sputum production), chest X-rays, and cultures.

Some people who experience pneumonia during their hospitalization will be left with long-term damage to their lungs. Damage may include chronic collapse of one or more lobes of the lung due to atelectasis, and stiffening of the lungs (fibrosis), which makes breathing much more difficult. The result is an inability to fully expand the lungs that can lead to more atelectasis, which can lead to recurrent infections, and subsequently, frequent rehospitalization—a vicious cycle. The best treatment is strengthening the muscles that help you breathe. Fortunately, there's a simple tool called an incentive spirometer that allows you to do that—provided you use it! (More about that on page 170.)

Ventilator-associated pneumonia (VAP) is a common and serious problem for people with severe ANI. To prevent VAP, doctors take a basic and effective approach: 1) elevating the head of the bed more than 30 degrees to keep bacteria from migrating into the lungs; 2) decreasing sedation to allow patients to follow commands and staff to evaluate readiness to remove the breathing tube; 3) administering frequent oral care to remove bacteria-containing plaques; 4) using endotracheal tubes that facilitate suctioning of secretions; and 5) making patients get out of bed as soon as possible, even while still attached to the ventilator.

Getting off the ventilator (extubation): Once you are placed on a ventilator, you enter a different level of complexity in terms of your medical care, and you may need a ventilator long enough that it becomes part of your chronic care. There is a three-step process to help you get off the ventilator and return to breathing on your own. It consists of readiness testing, weaning, and extubation.

A number of criteria are used to assess readiness. These include improvement in the underlying illness and adequate oxygen in the blood while breathing on your own. Weaning involves decreasing the assistance that the ventilator provides so that you need to do a greater amount of breathing on your own. A common approach is to use the spontaneous breathing test every day. The test consists of stopping the ventilator for thirty minutes while maintaining pressure to keep your airways open and oxygen below 40 percent. A successful breathing test includes a breathing rate less than 35 breaths per minute, stable vital signs, and blood oxygen saturation greater than 90 percent. If you fail the test, the underlying problem should be identified and treated more aggressively. If you pass the test, you are ready to start the extubation process as long as your underlying condition is improving, you have a strong cough, can handle your secretions, and are mentally alert. After extubation, you should be closely monitored for at least twenty-four hours.

Bronchospasm is the suddenly contraction of the muscles that line the airways, which forces the airways to close. It's caused by persistent inflammation around the smaller airways in the lung. The inflammatory cells secrete substances that stimulate the smooth muscle cells in the airways to contract suddenly (a spasm). If enough airways close at the same time, lung failure can occur. If you're on a ventilator, bronchospasm will make it harder for air to get into all parts of the lung, leading to lung collapse. Treatment is directed at the underlying problems, which are inflammation and spasms. Inflammation is best treated with antibiotics, which kill the bacteria and remove the bacterial toxins that attract inflammatory cells. Spasms are best treated with drugs that keep the airway muscles dilated (bronchodilators;

e.g., beta agonists like Albuterol), which are used in asthma and chronic obstructive pulmonary disease (COPD).

Tracheostomy: A tracheostomy is simply an opening into your trachea. It allows mechanical ventilation without an endotracheal tube (the clear plastic tube in the mouth or nose when on a ventilator). A tracheostomy is performed when there's a high likelihood that you will need mechanical ventilation for more than ten days after hospital admission. A tracheostomy is easier to breathe through than an endotracheal tube, much more comfortable, and makes it easier to talk and suction out secretions.

For me, all of these advantages were worth the surgery. I wanted to start physical therapy as soon as possible, and a tracheostomy allowed me to do that. This meant I could be extubated twenty-one days after my admission to the hospital. Some people may not be able to be weaned off the ventilator even with a tracheostomy, but many can strengthen their respiratory effort without mechanical ventilation.

CPAP (continuous-positive airway pressure): If you don't need ICU care and a ventilator but require some breathing support, there are noninvasive CPAP machines that assist breathing. These devices supply continuous positive airway pressure that keeps airways open via a mouthpiece or mask and oxygen or air as needed. They have a smaller chance of bacterial entry than ventilators and therefore result in fewer respiratory infections. Because no tracheostomy is needed, these devices also are much more comfortable.

Sleep apnea: Sleep apnea is a common condition characterized by periods of no breathing—for up to thirty seconds at a time—repeatedly throughout the night. Untreated, sleep apnea increases risk of stroke, heart attack, erectile dysfunction, and high blood pressure; it also causes daytime sleepiness, lethargy, anxiety, and fatigue. The factors that can cause sleep apnea include a dysfunctional ANS, respiratory muscle weakness, obesity, drugs that reduce spasticity by relaxing muscles, and sleeping on your back rather than your side. Sleep apnea is treated with devices such as CPAP.

Long-Term Treatments to Improve Lung Health

To combat any lung problems, it's a good idea to improve your breathing effort. There are several therapies that can strengthen your breathing.

SCI and the Diaphragm

The diaphragm and other muscles associated with respiration are not usually affected by stroke or TBI, but SCI patients with injuries at C5 or higher lack innervation of the diaphragm and usually require a ventilator. Even when SCI occurs at lower cervical levels or in the mid-thoracic levels, coordination of breathing will be impaired, usually for a few months, but sometimes permanently. This makes it difficult to take a deep breath and exhale forcefully, which significantly impairs your ability to cough. Poor cough makes you more prone to atelectasis, aspiration, and difficulty clearing secretions.

Exercise: Like all muscles, your respiratory muscles can increase in strength and stamina with exercise. Strengthening them will enable you to do more in rehab and at home, but it's equally important to improve your ability to cough and clear secretions, which decreases infections and the incidence of pneumonia. The most popular and effective respiratory muscle training device is the incentive spirometer (Figure 24). It's a simple plastic device that does not require a battery or electricity. You will likely be given one in the hospital—ask for one if you're not.

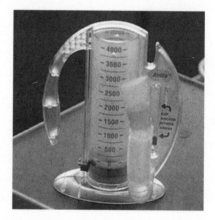

Figure 24. Incentive spirometer

To use the spirometer, hold the mouthpiece between your lips and take a long, deep inhale, making the little ball move to the highest possible position and *holding it there* as you continue to inhale for an increasing length of time (usually starting with fifteen seconds). When you can no longer continue the inhale, remove the mouthpiece and hold your breath for three seconds before making a deep, strong exhale. Repeat this exercise throughout the day for the prescribed number of repetitions.

It may be surprisingly difficult, at first, to get the little ball to where it should be; this exercise really makes your breathing muscles work hard! But with regular use, the incentive spirometer is highly effective and an excellent way to improve your lung function and avoid pneumonia. Once you're able, your physical therapist will likely have you performing a cardiovascular exercise that increases your respiratory rate and heart rate. And it's very important to strengthen your abdominal muscles, which can further assist with your inhalation. Don't forget exhalation either, because the ability to cough is partly dependent on the elastic recoil of your rib cage and diaphragm. To improve this elasticity, perform incentive spirometry and core-stretching exercises.

Pacing electrode: A pacing electrode may be placed on your diaphragm to stimulate movement of your diaphragm, even if it isn't innervated. The electrode and its battery are surgically implanted, and the strength and frequency of pacing are adjusted to improve your breathing effort as measured by incentive spirometry. It's also common practice to perform pulmonary function tests if you have a pacing electrode. These tests measure the amount of air you can hold in your lungs, the rate at which they fill, and the speed and volume of an exhalation.

Vaccinations: Get the recommended vaccinations for pneumonia and a yearly influenza (flu) vaccination. I also strongly recommend that you get the COVID-19 vaccine, because COVID-19 carries serious risk of pneumonia and long term complications.

Dealing with Lung Secretions and Mucus

Mucolytics: Three types of mucolytic agents assist in clearing mucus from the lungs: 1) Expectorants increase airway water to help with mucus clearing; 2) Mucoregulators increase the movement of mucus via cough; 3) Mucokinetics suppress the mechanisms causing excess mucus secretion. Your doctor will prescribe one or more of these medicines. It's also important to drink adequate water to thin mucus naturally.

Percussion: Percussion (slapping the back or chest) can physically mobilize and break apart mucus plugs. A caregiver can tap with fingers or an open hand where they hear no breath sounds. To help you cough the mucus out, an assistant can push upward on your stomach at the same time you cough to strengthen the force of air movement.

Posture and movement: To move mucus from the bottom of the lungs to airways higher up where it is easier to cough it out, you can perform postural drainage, which uses gravity. This is best done in a hospital bed by raising the feet and lowering the head for 15 to 20 minutes. It also helps if you increase movement by turning over in bed, or by standing up (with assistance) and moving back and forth.

Everything You Need to Know

After your injury, you're more susceptible to pneumonia, which is a leading cause of death. A small number of people will require a ventilator during their hospitalization.

- Once you're on the ventilator, there is a protocol to test your readiness to be weaned off the ventilator and extubated.

- Your best strategy to maintain healthy lungs is to avoid pneumonia with prevention. This begins in the hospital and continues after discharge. You should get the yearly influenza vaccine as well as the appropriate COVID-19 vaccine.

- Strengthen the muscles that help you breathe by using an incentive spirometer daily, and by performing cardiovascular exercise (with your doctor's approval) at least three times a week.

- If you snore, request a sleep study; if it reveals sleep apnea, be vigilant about using the CPAP mask and machine every night.

- If you smoke, quit! And stay away from smokers; second-hand smoke damages your lungs and can increase the likelihood of pneumonia.

13

Skin Health:
Preventing Pressure Ulcers

AFTER MY INJURY, I was unable to move and therefore at high risk for developing pressure ulcers. As a doctor, I knew how serious they were. And that knowledge worked—to this day, I've never developed a pressure ulcer. If you're partially or completely paralyzed in any limb, or lack sensation, you are at risk for developing a pressure ulcer. If you lack sensation, you can't tell when your skin begins to hurt. In fact, any time you spend extended periods of time in one position without moving, putting pressure on a vulnerable part of your body for a prolonged amount of time, you are susceptible to a pressure ulcer. For example, if you cross your legs in bed at night and have one ankle or knee resting on another ankle or knee for eight hours, you may develop a pressure ulcer. In this chapter, you'll learn how to maintain healthy skin and avoid pressure ulcers, because prevention is the best medicine.

What Is a Pressure Ulcer?

Pressure ulcers—also called bedsores, decubitus ulcers, and pressure sores—are areas where the skin breaks down (actually, it dies) due to a lack of oxygen. This happens when there are high levels of prolonged pressure, which can occur when you are sitting or lying for several hours without moving. Sustained pressure on places such as your tailbone and pelvis can decrease blood flow to deeper skin layers, leading to death of skin cells, infection, and ulcers.

How to Recognize Pressure Ulcers

The earliest appearance of a pressure ulcer is usually a red spot that does not blanch (return to a normal flesh color) after being pressed. Press on the red or dark area with your finger. The area should turn white if you have a lighter skin tone or become lighter than your normal skin color if you have darker skin. If, when you remove the pressure, the area returns to a red or dark color within a few seconds (indicating good blood flow), the discoloration is *not* a pressure ulcer. If the area stays lightened, the blood flow has been impaired and damage has begun. It's important to perform this test for any discoloration, even if it's as small as a quarter-inch in diameter, because an ulcer is like an iceberg. Beneath the red area may be a large sack of fluid that is much bigger than what you can see.

Stages and Treatment: Pressure ulcers are classified in four stages based on the ulcer surface area, depth, edges, tunneling, undermining, exudate type, and amount of dead tissue (Figure 25).

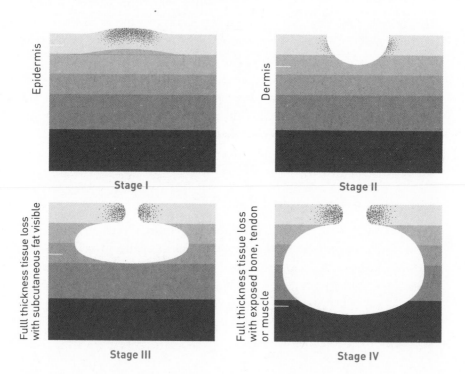

Figure 25. Stages of pressure ulcers

- **Stage I:** Intact skin that is red but does not blanch in a localized area, usually over a bony prominence. (Note: Stage I pressure ulcers may be difficult to detect in people who have darkly pigmented skin; ask your doctor or nurse to help you identify what a stage I pressure would look like on you.) Treatment: See your doctor and take all pressure off the site. Healing time is about three days.

- **Stage II:** An obvious loss of skin that has become a shallow, open ulcer with a red or pink wound bed or that has a fluid-filled blister. See your doctor *immediately*. Healing time is three days to three weeks.

- **Stage III:** Full-thickness skin loss; fat is visible but bone, tendon, or muscle are not exposed. There may be pieces of dead skin present. There may also be undermining and tunneling of the pressure ulcer. See your doctor *immediately*; you may be referred to a wound care specialist. Healing time ranges from one to three months.

- **Stage IV:** Full-thickness skin and tissue loss with exposed bone, tendon, or muscle. Dead skin or brown to black colored material (eschar) may be present in the wound. Stage IV ulcers can extend into muscle, tendon, or joint capsule, making bone infection (osteomyelitis) likely. Surgery is frequently required. Healing time ranges from three months to two years.

Causes and Risk Factors

There are four mechanisms that contribute to pressure ulcer development. Learning which situations in your daily life include them enables you to take precautions and to develop other approaches for tasks that are high-risk.

External pressure: The most common cause of pressure ulcers is something pushing against your skin with sufficient force and time to prevent blood flow to the tissue. Because bony prominences are hard and located near the skin surface, they are the most common sites where pressure causes ischemia (deficiency of blood flow) and hypoxia (deficiency of oxygen). The cells in the skin may start to die within ten minutes to two hours, depending on your nutritional state, blood flow to the affected skin (which is decreased in people with diabetes and peripheral vascular disease), and fluid in the skin (edema).

Friction: Friction damages the superficial blood vessels directly under the skin when you rub your skin against a surface repetitively. This can occur when you are being moved in bed or transferred onto a stretcher. When I'm pedaling on a stationary recumbent bike, I have to be careful that my shoulder blades don't rub against the seat back. If I rock too much from side to side, a blister can form on my back.

Shearing: Shearing occurs when your skin is moved more rapidly than the underlying tissue, causing it to separate. For example, when you're sitting up in bed, your skin may stick to the sheet, and when you slide down toward the foot of the bed, the movement can cause shearing. Shearing can also occur if you don't transfer properly and skid from your chair to the neighboring surface. Shearing disrupts the blood vessels between the skin, fat, and muscle.

Moisture: Sweat, urine, feces, and wound drainage increase skin friction and accelerate the damage done by pressure and shear. Prolonged exposure to moisture breaks down the skin's natural protective barrier, making it more likely to become infected. To avoid this problem, it's important to change dressings and clothes as soon as they get wet.

Risk Factors: There are more than one hundred risk factors for pressure ulcers, but the major ones include immobility, type 2 diabetes, peripheral vascular disease, poor nutrition, and low blood pressure. Additional factors are being over the age of seventy, smoking, dry skin, urinary and fecal incontinence, and a history of pressure ulcers.

How to Prevent Pressure Ulcers

Good news: 95 percent of all pressure ulcers are preventable!

Inspection: Pressure ulcers usually occur in areas of skin that lack sensation. Because you may not *feel* the problem, you and your caregiver should check your skin twice a day (in the morning and before you go to bed at night). Carefully inspect areas that are at the highest risk, which are places where the skin covers a bone, particularly the sacrum (lower back), coccyx (tailbone), ischium (the base of the buttocks, aka "sit bones"), trochanters (hip), knees, ankles, heels, toes, and bony areas of the feet. Inspect any areas of skin that are in contact with casts or braces, and bruises, especially if they're below your waist.

Pressure relief and redistribution: Pressure relief is simply moving or lifting yourself to take the pressure off the skin that has been under pressure, usually from sitting or lying in one position, so that blood can circulate. You'll need to shift throughout the day and night routinely so that it becomes a habit. Before you leave the hospital, your therapist will teach you how to do pressure relief.

The methods and timing of pressure relief depend on your injury and skin tolerance. On a manual wheelchair cushion, this usually means shifting your weight off bony prominences every fifteen to thirty minutes for a duration of at least thirty to ninety seconds; a single "pushup" from a standard wheelchair is *not* adequate to prevent pressure ulcers; you'll need to do several. On an electric chair, there should be a tilt function that enables you to offload weight from your sacrum, coccyx, and ischium every two hours. On a mattress, you'll need to roll over every two to four hours; set a timer with an alarm to remind yourself.

Use pillows and foam pads (not folded towels or blankets) to protect bony areas. No two skin surfaces with bone underneath (especially knees and ankles) should ever rest against each other as you sleep. If you're at high risk, your doctor may prescribe a special bed or cushion that distributes the pressure against your skin so that there are no high-pressure spots. There are also pressure-mapping mats that can be used to measure the pressure your body exerts against your bed or your chair cushion. Using that information, equipment specialists can adjust the mattress and cushion to eliminate the high-pressure spots.

Skin hygiene: It's essential to keep your skin clean and dry. Bathe daily with mild, non-abrasive soap and rinse and dry your skin thoroughly. If you've leaked stool or urine, immediately wash and dry your skin. Avoid skin sanitizers that have alcohol, as well as antibacterial soaps. Don't use any powders. Dry skin can be a significant problem, particularly on the lower legs, if you have edema. Be sure to keep your skin moist with the daily application of a body lotion approved by your doctor.

Support surfaces: There are three common support surfaces for wheelchair seat cushions and mattresses: foam, gel, and air-filled. There are pros and cons for each type of support. Foam is the least expensive but also the least durable, and it can't be adjusted. Gel conforms to your body and maintains an even pressure over bony prominences, but it doesn't breathe and is hotter and more likely to allow moisture to develop. It's also heavier than air or foam supports. Air cushions consist of soft, flexible air-filled containers called cells that are connected by small channels, which are adjusted by inflating them with varying amounts of air. A more expensive air cushion for both bed and wheelchair is one in which the pressure changes regularly using multiple air chambers that are alternately pumped up and down. While these pressure-redistributing support surfaces may seem like the best choice, there are no large studies confirming a significant improvement. There are also mattresses in which an air pump blows a continuous flow of air under the entire support surface. These are excellent at distributing pressure, but the air flow may make you feel cold. (More on this in chapter 15.)

Nutrition: Adequate intake of protein and calories is important to prevent pressure ulcers, because people who have less muscle and fat to protect the areas covering the bone are at higher risk. Skin health depends on making keratin, the major protein that comprises skin, which is highly dependent on diet. If you develop a pressure ulcer, consider seeing a nutritionist to make sure that your diet is sufficient for ulcer prevention. The standard recommendation is a protein intake of 1.2 to 1.5 gm/kg body weight daily.[1] If the ulcer is stage III or IV, the fluid that drains from it will have high levels of protein and sugars, so your intake of high-quality protein and nutrient-rich calories should be increased as well. Don't waste your money on supplements; there are none that have shown a benefit for healing pressure ulcers.

Treating Pressure Ulcers

When you and your doctor make a decision regarding medical or surgical treatment for an ulcer, it will be helpful to consider the overall size and composition of the pressure ulcer.

Principles of treatment: Most pressure ulcers should be treated medically, with surgery being a last resort. The key to effective treatment is recognizing any underlying medical conditions (like type 2 diabetes) and treating those conditions intensively, as well as improving nutrition, relieving pressure and shear force, keeping the wound moist and covered, and helping the body get rid of dead skin and tissue with debridement.

Medical Therapy

Debridement (removal of tissue): In most cases, dead tissue should be removed, because it provides an ideal place for bacteria to grow. As your wound care specialist will explain, there are several ways to remove dead tissue, starting with your body's own system, which is called autolytic debridement. Debriding the ulcer requires multiple approaches which may include dressings that selectively remove dead tissue, cleaning with mildly abrasive bactericidal soap, use of a whirlpool to warm the ulcer and improve blood flow while agitating dead tissue away, and negative pressure to suck the dead tissue away and increase blood flow.

Dressings: Despite many studies, it's unclear which topical agent or dressing is best for treating pressure ulcers. Protease-containing dressings, antimicrobial drug dressings (containing antibiotics or metals like zinc and silver), foam dressings, hydrogel dressings, and collagenase ointment may be better for healing than plain gauze, because they more rapidly and selectively remove dead tissue. Some of them also kill bacteria (antibiotics) or prevent proliferation (zinc and silver).

Antibiotics: The jury is still out on whether antibiotics improve healing of pressure ulcers. This is likely due to the fact that poor blood vessel supply limits penetration of the antibiotics into the dead tissue where the bacteria are growing. But there's an *undisputed* role for antibiotics when the bacteria invade the bone, muscle, or—even worse—the bloodstream.

Surgical Therapy

Surgical debridement is the fastest method of removing dead tissue. A drawback to this approach (compared to autolytic debridement, your body's ability to rid itself of the dead tissue), is that it causes more damage to underlying *healthy* tissue, which increases the size of the ulcer. Stage III and IV pressure ulcers often require surgical intervention because of their high rate of recurrence and the length of time necessary for medical therapy to work (three months to two years). During this time, you are confined to your bed every day!

Surgery is the best option when the ulcer has tunneled into underlying tissue, especially bone and muscle, since medical therapy cannot reach deeper infections. Increasingly, closure after surgery uses skin grafts. In particular, skin "flaps" that contain their own blood supply are used, because they bring oxygen and white blood cells to fight the infection as well as protecting the underlying wound from contamination. The need for pressure relief and bedrest is even more critical after surgery, to allow the graft to join with the debrided skin and tissue and revitalize the ulcerated tissue.

Everything You Need to Know

Pressure ulcers are a serious threat to your health and recovery. You're at risk if you spend most of your day in a wheelchair or in bed. You can avoid pressure ulcers by following these proven prevention steps:

- Check your skin twice daily (and have someone else check the parts of your body you can't see) for signs of pressure ulcers.

- Notify your doctor as soon as you find what you believe may be a pressure ulcer.

- Avoid staying in the same seated or prone position for long periods of time.

- Invest in quality pressure-relieving support cushions, mattresses, and devices.

- Eat a nutritious diet.

- Keep your skin clean, dry, and properly moisturized.

14

Muscle, Bone, and Joint Health

PRIOR TO MY INJURY, I exercised vigorously for one hour every day. My good health helped me after my injury; during my ten days in the ICU, unable to move, I lost five percent of my muscle mass. I'm positive that the health of my body at the time of my injury and my love of physically demanding workouts were (and continue to be) instrumental in my recovery.

Don't get me wrong—after my accident, I was paralyzed. The effort it has taken to get to where I am today has been significant. From the moment it began, my physical therapy was excruciatingly difficult and left me completely exhausted. All these years later, PT is still a challenging part of my life, but I know the benefits are worth the effort and, yes, the pain. Making my muscles work hard helps my heart, my lungs, my bones and joints, and even my brain. It also means I can be as independent as possible, which improves my quality of life. And all of that means greater longevity.

Your ability to exercise will be a fundamental component of successful functional recovery, and also for maintaining muscle mass and bone density. If you're paralyzed and unable to move, your muscles and bones waste away, making exercise difficult, which sets in motion a vicious cycle. But the good news is that you can break that cycle. Existing technologies that move paralyzed limbs, such as functional electrical stimulation (Figure 26; see page 184), body weight support and balance systems, robots, and exoskeletons (Figures 27–29; see pages 185–186), are useful. There are also less expensive ways to support your muscle and bone health, depending on the severity of your injury. Let's take a look.

Muscle Function

Skeletal muscles are made up of bundles of muscle cells, or fibers; most skeletal muscles are attached to bones by tendons. For a muscle to move, a signal must be transmitted from the top of your brain (the motor cortex) down the spinal cord in a neuron. The neurons leave the spinal cord as a nerve fiber, and then spread out over the muscle to cause it to contract. This combination of motor neuron and the muscle fibers that it innervates is called the motor unit. After an ANI, the muscle motor unit undergoes profound changes due to death of the motor neurons in the brain or spinal cord that cause paralysis.

If your injury has left you paralyzed, you may feel a desire to move your limbs and use them to be independent. But, depending on your injury, it can take weeks to months before nerves can regrow from the site of injury to the muscle. As more nerves connect with muscle, the muscle gains strength. It can do this in two different ways. First, in a process called hypertrophy, each muscle fiber can grow larger to do the work of two or more fibers that are not innervated. Second, dormant cells in the muscle, called satellite cells, can be stimulated to make a new muscle cell, which is then incorporated into the existing muscle. The nerve itself can promote muscle growth by extending new branches to neighboring motor neurons. This recruits more muscles that lack their own innervation. When a muscle grows bigger, it grows stronger.

Muscle Atrophy

Immobility: Your muscles begin to shrink in size by 0.5 percent per day when you stop using them due to denervation or injury. I was immobile for one-and-a-half months before I could move my legs. By then, I had lost fifteen pounds—10 percent of my body weight. If the loss had been muscle only, that wouldn't have been so bad, but when muscle atrophies, it's usually replaced by fat. So I had actually lost 15 to 20 percent of my muscle mass. "Use it or lose it" is especially true when it comes to your muscles, which is why physical therapy carefully exercises your muscles, even when you're unable to move them voluntarily.

Central nervous system damage: The death of neurons in the brain or spinal cord can cause significant muscle atrophy. Usually, the atrophy is limited to the paralyzed limb, but if you've suffered sufficient brain damage, there can be widespread muscle atrophy—in your arms, core, and legs—without paralysis.

Peripheral nervous system damage: There can also be damage to nerves in the peripheral nervous system, outside the spinal cord. When I fell from my bike and hit my head, I put out my right arm to lessen the impact. But I overextended it, and the nerves in that armpit (the brachial plexus) were stretched and damaged. This injury probably contributed to some of the muscle atrophy in my right arm, which is now only 25 percent as strong as my left arm. So it's important that your doctors look for peripheral nerve damage, which can result from stretching, compression, or direct trauma. Sometimes, it's possible to stretch, exercise, and massage (using myofascial techniques) the affected limb to release the nerve. In other instances, a surgical repair is necessary.

Strengthening Muscle

To regain your strength and coordination, you may need to combine multiple therapies in a program designed expressly for you. The program may include range-of-motion work, strengthening, functional training, patient and family education, and equipment training. For muscle strengthening, your program may include some or all of the following: good nutrition (increased protein, especially leucine, and sufficient calories), independent physical activity (resistance and weight training and cardiovascular exercise), assisted physical activity using functional electrical stimulation (FES; Figure 26), body weight support systems (including robots and exoskeletons); and drugs such as testosterone and anabolic steroids (androgens such as methandrostenolone, also known as performance-enhancing drugs or PEDs).

Use it or lose it: Activity-based therapies (ABT) have great potential to improve motor function. These activities include locomotor training, FES, and task-specific training. All of these interventions are intended to stimulate the nervous system and optimize functional recovery. Recovery can be via neuroplasticity (reorganization of the nervous system and recruitment of nerve pathways not used routinely) or activity-based programs, which have benefits beyond improved motor function, including improvements in cardiac function, bone density, muscle mass, and glucose metabolism. After walking daily using my platform walker for up to fifteen minutes at a time, I've increased the pressure sensation in my feet, lumbar, and thoracic regions.

Much of the work in activity-based programs is performed by walking with assistance: treadmill walking with therapist assistance and body weight support (Figure 27), overground walking with only body weight support (e.g., Hocoma Andago, Figure 28A); robot treadmill walking with body weight support (e.g., Hocoma Lokomat, Figure 28B); and overground walking with exoskeletons, which are a type of robot with balance and body weight support in one unit (e.g., ReWalk exoskeletons Figures 29A & B). Results from a number of studies of ABT have shown improvements in trunk control, endurance, walking speed, balance, and ability to perform activities of daily living. For people with upper-extremity weakness, the use of robots to move and strengthen the upper extremities can be helpful. For a year, I used the BIONIK InMotion robot (see pages 47–48) for one-hour sessions three times a week and increased my upper-extremity strength and coordination significantly.

There are four main ways ABT helps in moving the lower extremities:

1. **Functional electrical stimulation** (FES; Figure 26) uses electrodes to deliver small voltage shocks to stimulate dormant nerves and artificially cause muscle contraction. It is most commonly configured to enable bicycle pedaling, because it can be done by you alone for periods of time up to one hour.

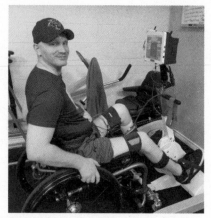

Figure 26. Functional electrical stimulation (FES)

2. **The Lokomat treadmill** (Figure 27) uses two therapists who each move one leg in a coordinated manner to stimulate a normal gait. In some people, who are able to perform intensive therapy for several months, paralyzed limbs can recover strength and coordinated movement, so the person may walk independently.[1]

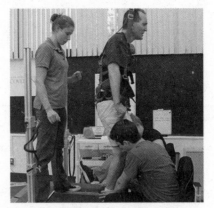

Figure 27. Treadmill locomotor training

3. **Suspension systems,** like the Hocoma Andago, or a suspension system plus powered movement like the robotic Hocoma Lokomat (Figure 28), provide weight support and balance; thereby enabling you to practice walking overground and turning.

A   B

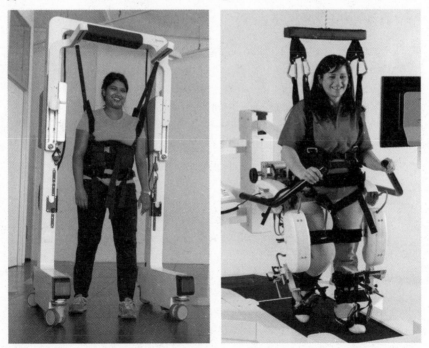

Figure 28. Locomotion devices: A. Hocoma Andago, and B. Hocoma Lokomat.

A   B

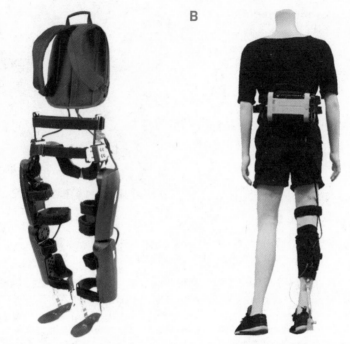

Figure 29. Robots: A. ReWalk Personal 6.0 Exoskeleton, and B. ReWalk ReStore Exosuit

4. **Robots** like the ReWalk Personal (Figure 29A) and the ReWalk ReStore Exosuit (Figure 29B) provide body weight support and balance, in addition to robot-assisted lower extremity movement, which permits independent walking on a treadmill or overground for people who have serious deficits in walking due to motor and/or sensory loss. In the future, I believe that locally implanted epidural electrical stimulators (or eventually transcutaneous electrical stimulators) will enable independent walking by combining the best features of current technology (see chapter 19). Powered exoskeletons use a combination of electric motors, hydraulics, and gyroscopes to enable the wearer to move with more strength and control.

There are several models available, but none of them have become simple enough to put on, take off, and use to become the preferred method for walking. That said, they are excellent devices (but expensive) for strengthening your limbs and core. Further advances in materials for construction and batteries will likely make them more useful in the future. But for now, even the psychological benefits of being able to stand up and walk are tremendous. More on exoskeletons on page 210.

Common Musculoskeletal Overuse Injuries

Upper Limb and Shoulder

Rotator cuff injury: The rotator cuff, tendons that keep the upper arm bone (humerus) in place, is designed to give you the greatest freedom of motion—it's how you scratch your back, brush your hair, or reach for something above your head. The rotator cuff is not, however, designed for moving heavy objects or repetitive motions. Consequently, any person with ANI is at risk in the long term for damaging their rotator cuff. This occurs most frequently in manual wheelchair users but can occur in anyone who has weakness of the muscles that make up the rotator cuff. For example, my rotator cuff screams "ouch" after I spend an hour using my right arm to control the computer mouse, and when I use it to steer the bike while cycling. It could happen easily when you are carrying a water pitcher, stirring batter while cooking, or reaching up into a cabinet to get a dish or glass.

Pushing a manual wheelchair using your triceps and your rotator cuff places an unnatural burden on them. Over time, the muscles atrophy and the tendons fray, making them susceptible to breakage. The constant wear and tear also lead to inflammation and pain. Fortunately, there are several exercises that will strengthen these muscles. It is helpful to adjust your wheelchair to make pushing as efficient as possible, as is purchasing the lightest chair possible (see page 202). The chair's setup should position the rear axle as far forward as it can go, and seating should be adjusted to maintain optimal posture.

Learn the early signs of rotator cuff injury so that you can switch (temporarily) from a manual wheelchair to an electric modified third wheel (see page 203) or power wheelchair, and allow your shoulders to rest and heal. Some new wheelchairs have electric motors in the hubs of the wheels that allow you to use them as manual power-driven. If you have shoulder problems and use a manual wheelchair, investigate these chairs so that you have the option to switch to power or electric-assist as needed.

Frozen shoulder: Frozen shoulder happens when the muscles of the shoulder are kept immobile due to paralysis or pain. The muscles shorten, inflammation occurs, and the tissues around the head of your shoulder bone (humerus) become attached by weblike strands of fibrotic tissue that cause extreme stiffness and loss of range of motion (adhesive capsulitis). This process dramatically decreases the shoulder's range of motion, especially when you try to rotate your arm in and out. The best treatment for frozen shoulder is to prevent it by maintaining movement. Once frozen shoulder occurs, anti-inflammatory drugs in combination with stretching and physical therapy can help improve and restore range of motion.

Hand, Wrist, and Elbow

Carpal tunnel syndrome (CTS): CTS is the most common overuse injury, affecting 40 to 65 percent of wheelchair users. The causes of the repetitive stress are transfers, weight shifts, and pushing the wheelchair. The symptoms are weakness and numbness of the hand, a worsening of symptoms while sleeping, and slight improvement by shaking the wrist.

CTS is diagnosed by electromyography (EMG). Treatment is usually conservative and includes using padded gloves to push your wheelchair, wearing a splint while you sleep at night to stretch the wrist, over-the-counter anti-inflammatory drugs, and, occasionally, steroid injections. If, after three months of these treatments, the pain is still debilitating, you may consider surgery. Surgery is performed under local anesthetic and has high success rates, but the inability to use your hand during the recovery period may be difficult, as you will need more help with your everyday tasks. And you'll need to use an electric wheelchair while you recover.

Ulnar nerve compression (elbow): Compression of the ulnar nerve (commonly called "hitting your funny bone") due to entrapment at the elbow is the second most common peripheral nerve problem, affecting 25 to 45 percent of wheelchair users. The symptoms are shooting pain down your forearm and numbness of the little and ring fingers. Treatment is basic: Avoid situations that put pressure on the inner part of your elbow (such as resting your arm on your armrest or table) or keeping your elbow flexed for long periods of time.

Lateral (tennis elbow) and medial (flexor tendonitis) epicondylitis: The bumps on the underside of your elbow are called the epicondyles. Wheelchair users who grip their rims too hard or are not sitting properly may develop lateral epicondylitis (pain and tenderness on the outer side of the elbow). You can also overuse the flexor pronator muscle by extending the wrist too high when pushing your wheelchair, which causes pain on the inner side of the elbow (this is not uncommon when your wrist and finger strength are weak, which is typical of tetraplegics). Treatment for either condition is improving your wheelchair technique, applying an ice pack to the painful area, stretching and strengthening the muscles with physical therapy, steroid injections, and using an electric wheelchair when necessary.

Musculoskeletal Complications

Osteoporosis: Osteoporosis means your bones have lost density, making them weaker and more breakable. There are generally no symptoms; all too often osteoporosis is diagnosed after even a minor fall results in a broken bone. Bone weakening occurs primarily in paralyzed limbs because of lack of use and decreased weight-bearing. Osteoporosis is diagnosed with a bone density scan.

People with ANI have rapid loss of bone density.[2] Within two years, 60 percent will have developed osteoporosis; 20 percent will have mild bone density loss (osteopenia), and 20 percent will remain in the normal range. Over a fifteen-year period, 40 percent of people with ANI will have a fracture. Bones in regions of complex regional pain syndrome (CRPS) show increased osteoporosis. For example, the bones in my right forearm, which is where I have CRPS, have lost twice as much bone density as any other bones in my body.

Lifestyle changes are the first step in addressing osteoporosis. Good nutrition with adequate intake of calcium and vitamin D; weight-bearing exercise; smoking cessation; counseling on fall prevention; and avoidance of heavy alcohol use all help you limit bone thinning and fractures. Avoid, if possible, drugs that increase bone loss, such as certain steroids. Weight-bearing therapies, including the use of a standing frame, FES (which only works if maintained for a prolonged period of time), exercise, and whole-body vibration platforms can all help strengthen bone and limit loss of density.

Bisphosphonates are medications that inhibit bone resorption (loss of bone mass) and weakening. They are the most frequently prescribed drugs because of their efficacy, low cost, and safety. In a review of many trials of people with osteoporosis, bisphosphonates reduced the risk of fracture by 40 to 60 percent. Your doctor can discuss the best options for you.

Osteoarthritis (OA): OA is a common condition as we age. It causes joint pain and a subsequent reduction in activities, which leads to a loss of range of motion, causing functional impairment—a domino effect. OA affects both large joints (knee, hip, shoulder) and small joints (fingers and wrist). Consequently, it causes difficulty walking, bending over, reaching overhead, performing tasks with your hands such as opening a jar, knitting, cooking, even opening a letter. The upper extremity, particularly the shoulder joint, is frequently affected by osteoarthritis. OA of the knee, hip, and shoulder is common in all three ANIs because there is frequently an imbalance, created by different sensory and motor abilities on one side of your body. This is particularly common if you use a cane or have use of only one arm and hand, making the limb susceptible to OA from overuse. Treatment of OA should be conservative, starting with therapy to improve range of motion; nonsteroidal anti-inflammatory drugs such as ibuprofen; and exercise of muscles to prevent disuse atrophy.

Osteomyelitis: Most commonly the result of a pressure ulcer that has extended into the underlying bone, osteomyelitis should be considered a non–healing stage IV pressure ulcer. It's best diagnosed with a bone scan or MRI. Frequently, bone biopsy is needed to identify the bacteria causing it. Treatment is administration of intravenous antibiotics for six to twelve weeks. If healing is still delayed after antibiotics, the bone may need to be removed, especially if there's evidence of systemic spread of the infection.

Radiculopathy and Myelopathy: Osteoarthritis-associated inflammation can lead to radiculopathy. In a radiculopathy, a nerve is pinched as it exits the spinal cord through a narrowed hole (foramen) in the vertebrae. The most common location is in the neck, especially at the sixth and seventh vertebrae, which is also one of the most common sites for SCI. Over time, bone spurs can further obstruct the foramen. When a radiculopathy occurs months to years after your injury, it can be frightening because your first thought may be that something has "gone wrong" in your brain or spinal cord. The major symptoms are pain and muscle weakness (myelopathy).

Diagnosis is usually made with an X-ray of the neck or a CT scan and electromyography (EMG). EMG measures the speed of the nerve impulse from the brain to the affected muscle. It can determine whether the problem is in the brain or in nerves outside the spinal cord; the latter is much more common. Treatment is conservative, including stretching for range of motion, bed rest, and physical therapy. For pain, nonsteroidal anti-inflammatory drugs are usually prescribed. There is also evidence that chiropractic treatment is helpful, but only for neck pain that is not due to a radiculopathy but is caused by chronic musculoskeletal problems.[3] Usually, the pain and weakness resolve after four to eight weeks. If symptoms continue, you may require additional testing with MRI to rule out other causes.

SCI-Specific Musculoskeletal Problems

Post-operative spine degeneration: Many people will require an operation to stabilize their spine. In my case, I had surgery to fuse my vertebrae from C3 to C5. As a result, I have a decreased range of motion for movements such as spinal flexion, extension, and rotation. More important, the fused vertebrae act like a lever and push against the adjacent vertebrae, especially the lower ones (C6 to T1 in my case). This accelerates the normal process of wear and tear that causes degeneration of the disc and erosion of the vertebrae.

Over many years, this can lead to new neurologic deficits and a disease called neuropathic spinal arthropathy. Because this process can worsen pain as well as motor and sensory function, you should have yearly exams to document your muscle strength and sensation. The diagnosis is best made by CT scan, which can show narrowing of vertebral discs and erosion of parts of the vertebrae. Unfortunately, there aren't any particularly good treatments for neuropathic spinal arthropathy. But physical therapy to strengthen the muscles can be helpful, and so can exercises to increase range of motion. These activities can sometimes worsen pain, in which case immobilizing the neck is recommended using a custom fitted brace. Surgery to fuse damaged vertebrae will likely decrease pain, but this can lead to further damage of your spine by the same arthropathy process.

Heterotopic ossification: Heterotopic ossification is the development of bone deposits in soft (nonskeletal) tissue, primarily around the hip and knee joints. It occurs in many people with SCI and some with TBI. It can develop within days following the injury. In most cases, heterotopic ossification causes no significant physical limitations, but it can limit joint motion, cause swelling, or increase spasticity in the leg. In rare situations, drugs will need to be prescribed and surgery is sometimes necessary.

Loss of muscle mass (sarcopenia): From ages forty to eighty, the average American experiences a 35 percent decrease in total muscle and bone mass. This loss is called sarcopenia and is accompanied by decreased muscle strength. There are many causes, including decreased physical activity due to weakness, chronic pain, and fatigue; loss of muscle innervation, which is necessary to stimulate muscle contraction and promote muscle cell survival, repair, and regeneration; decreased caloric intake (especially protein); vitamin D deficiency; and decreased production of growth hormone and testosterone. Two ways to address the problem, supported by current studies, are: 1) exercise, which has been shown to increase muscle mass when weights are used in the upper extremity and sit-to-stand and gait training are used for the lower extremity[4]; and 2) adding protein to your diet in the form of fish, certain amino acids (e.g., leucine), and vitamin D for people with confirmed deficiency.[5] Speak with a nutritionist for expert advice on the best dietary and supplement options for you.

Everything You Need to Know

Your bone and muscle health are integral to your level of functioning and independent living. Strong muscles and bones are also key to longevity.

After your injury, you may experience significant bone and muscle loss. Work with your doctor and physical therapy team to ensure that you're doing all you can to maintain and even increase muscle mass and bone density. To the extent that you are able:

- Include weight-bearing exercise at least three times a week as part of your PT.

- Be sure your diet includes enough protein.

- Learn adaptive techniques that will protect you from rotator cuff injury, carpal tunnel syndrome, and other common conditions to which your injury has made you more vulnerable.

- Take advantage of the latest technologies when they can help you, such as robotic-assisted exercise therapy.

- When an injury occurs, start with the most conservative therapeutic approach and leave surgery as a last resort.

In addition to working with your physical therapy team to improve your muscle strength and bone density, investigate local groups of other people with ANI who participate in team sports or workouts such as swimming, bicycling, rowing, and basketball. You'll benefit from the camaraderie as well as the exercise.

PART 4

Enjoy a Rewarding and Meaningful Life

15

Miraculous Adaptations

How to Take Advantage of Life-Enhancing
Devices, Tools, and More

W HEN I WAS INJURED in 2009, there were very few adaptive devices for people with ANI to use a computer. But when the first iPad was released in 2010, it was transformative. Suddenly, with only limited use of my fingers and the voice dictation feature, I could read and write, just like I had with my computer before the accident.

Today, smartphones, tablets, and watches can open up the world for you at a very reasonable cost. They can help you interact with social networks, obtain information, read books, play games, and so much more. With smart home software, you can control your lights, security system, doors, heat and air-conditioning, entertainment system, and even your coffee maker. Even if your disability is medically complex, you can use these applications with voice recognition (usually standard) or head tracking and eye gaze technology (specialized and expensive) to control your environment, to assist you in your work (and play), and monitor your health.

There are many excellent devices that can have a tremendously positive impact on your quality of life. These include aids for every aspect of daily living: personal hygiene, dressing, eating, and transferring from your bed to your wheelchair, from your wheelchair to your car, and so on. There are tools to help you with communication: speaking, hearing, and seeing. And devices that help you walk: braces, walkers, and exoskeletons. There's a *huge* variety of wheelchairs and other mobility devices from which to choose that are designed for a variety of activities, including sports. There are even driverless cars (sort of!). Many of these adaptive devices and aids incorporate assistive technology (AT), which can be used to modify existing devices or to create new ones that enhance your safety and quality of life. You, your loved ones, and your health care team should work together to decide which devices would best suit your needs. Frequently, representatives from the companies that manufacture, sell, and service the devices can participate in the discussion; their expertise can be especially helpful. Whenever possible, ask for trial periods of high-ticket items. See information on these companies in the Resources section on page 283.

You or your caretaker should keep a notebook to help you compare the devices you're interested in. Among the important choices are mobility devices (wheelchairs, walkers, and scooters); walking-assistive devices (canes and crutches); beds and seat cushions; aids for daily living (reachers, handles, and grips); communication devices and sensory aids (hearing aids, talking boards, and Braille displays); adaptive computer equipment (ergonomic keyboards, hands-free mice, and screen readers); and wearable tracking devices for health and exercise (to monitor your heart rate, number of steps walked, and calories expended). Ask your therapist if you can demo expensive items for a week. Many rehabilitation centers have donated chairs and beds that you can test.

Simple Devices Can Make a Huge Difference

Early on in my rehabilitation, paralysis had so weakened my hands that I couldn't turn the pages of the paperbacks that friends had brought me. I was unable even to grasp a tissue and move it from right to left on my tray table when Patty, my physical therapist, instructed me to do so. I cried tears of despair and rage. Day after day in therapy, I very slowly strengthened my grip as I followed her instructions. Several months after she had started me on the hand exercises, Patty returned with a pencil and a book. She opened the book and laid it flat before me; holding the pencil with the eraser facing outward, she used it to grab the edge of a page and turn it over. Then, she handed the pencil to me. I grasped it with all my strength and finally turned a page. "I have my life back," I said, with tears overflowing, and we cried together. The pencil was one of many simple devices that I used in the beginning. Others included a grabber to reach objects outside of my range of motion; universal cuffs for handheld items; special forks, knives, and spoons with rings to make them easier to hold (see page 215); and a special cup for drinking that was covered with Dycem, an antibacterial, tacky material to make it easier to hold, and had a no-spill cap that kept it from pouring its contents out when I knocked it over.

In the future, there will be even more miraculous tools to choose from, some of which will be commercially available and others as part of clinical trials. Brain-computer interfaces (BCI), artificial vision, augmented speaking and hearing, and improved exoskeletons are all being tested in clinical trials. The brain-computer interface is the ultimate device. It allows a computer to "decode" your thoughts and translate them into an action via a robot, an exoskeleton, or your own limb, stimulated by implanted electrodes. Other assistive technologies include epidural electrical stimulation, robotics, and virtual reality (you'll find more about those technologies in chapter 19).

For all adaptive devices, it's critical that you have the necessary information to ask the right questions so that you can choose the correct device, with the proper modifications, for you. Talk with your health care team, particularly the rehab folks, the sales representatives for the devices, and fellow ANI survivors who have years of experience with specific devices. They will be a tremendous source of information for you.

Despite the advances in technology, one thing is as true today as it was at the time of my accident. The two most important adaptive devices are your bed and your wheelchair, if you'll be using one. Why? These two devices are where you'll spend up to 95 percent of your time, at least initially. So they must be the most functional, comfortable, safe, and personally appealing devices that you own.

Beds

Choosing the right bed is extremely important, because you will spend at least seven or eight hours in it every night. During that time, your body needs to recover from the rigors of the day. It's critical that the bed be comfortable and enable adequate blood flow to your skin and tissues, so that you do not develop pressure ulcers (see page 173). Many people choose to rent a hospital bed because it is an inexpensive choice (you can rent them by the month), and you can use the bed controller to change the height of your upper and lower body to find a comfortable position to sleep, eat meals, read, and watch television. One downside, however, is that the mattress material of hospital beds is firm and provides no redistribution of weight, which is essential to relieve pressure on your skin and tissues. As a result, you will be susceptible to pressure ulcers and must turn over every two to four hours to prevent them. If you're strong enough, you might be able to do this alone or use an overhead trapeze bar to help you turn. If you're unable to turn independently, you have three choices: have a companion or aide turn you; purchase a bed that can roll you over; or purchase a bed with excellent pressure relief, so that you can stay in one position all night.

The performance characteristics of beds may be widely different depending on the materials and assembly. Different mattress materials offer varying degrees of pressure relief and therefore different degrees of protection from pressure ulcers. Softer beds make transfers more difficult, but firmer beds may be more prone to causing high pressure on areas of the skin. When you are lying on your side, you are at risk of developing pressure ulcers in the tissue around the hip bones; when you are lying on your back, the risk of pressure ulcers is highest in the sacrum and heels. When you are lying on your back, keep the bed at a 30-degree elevation of the upper body to decrease pressure over bony prominences. Lying on your stomach distributes your weight naturally, but many people cannot tolerate this position. Pillows can be used to help to maintain your desired position and are particularly useful when lying on your side, where they can be placed between your knees to prevent your knees and ankles from touching each other and creating a high-pressure area.

There are five major types of mattress materials:

1. A regular mattress (e.g., a hospital bed) offers no significant benefits regarding pressure ulcer risk, and you must turn every two to four hours to relieve pressure on your skin and deep tissue.

2. Foam beds increase the support area and provide pressure reduction at a low cost, but the foam breaks down easily and will compress, making it less effective over time, so it must be replaced frequently.

3. Static flotation is usually the best combination for protection from pressure ulcers at a relatively low cost. The major types are "egg-crate" pressure mats, such as the ROHO cushion, in which groups of egg-shaped bubbles—usually 4 to 6 inches (10–15 cm) long by 12 to 16 inches (30–40 cm) wide—are assembled together to form a mattress. Each group of bubbles can be individually adjusted with more or less air to optimize pressure relief. I and many of my friends have found that the Sleep Number bed is a terrific static floatation device. You can adjust the pressure of the mattress over a wide range of settings, and it has the elevation capabilities of a hospital bed and independent

control of leg and torso positions. With the king-size bed, you and your sleeping partner can select individual pressure levels.

4. The highest level of support surface uses air flow to float your body without pressure points. These air flow beds are usually needed only when you are treating a pressure ulcer, because the air flow in the mattress feels cold, the pump for air movement is noisy, and they are expensive.

The type of sheets you use is important; heavy sheets (flannel and thick cotton) create shearing forces when you move, and they don't breathe as well as lighter sheets, making you hotter and increasing the risk of pressure ulcers. Bamboo sheets are the best choice because they allow your body to breathe easier and stay cooler.

Pillows need to maintain a level of support that prevents your head from tilting backward, which can occur spontaneously when you enter rapid eye movement (REM) sleep. If your pillow is too soft, you will put too much pressure on your neck, decreasing the area of your spinal canal and pinching your spinal cord, which may cause neuropathic pain and other symptoms.

Wheelchairs

Wheelchairs are usually the most expensive, important, custom-fitted, and complex assistive device that you will purchase. They are the preferred means of locomotion for paraplegics with normal upper body strength but paralyzed legs; people with TBI and stroke who have paralysis severe enough that they don't have the strength to walk long distances; or anyone with an ANI who has balance problems due to loss of sensation or damage to the cerebellum that makes them too unsteady to walk.

The thought of spending any time in a wheelchair can be depressing, so let me share these words from the United Spinal Association: *People are not confined to their wheelchairs—they are in fact liberated by their wheels.* For me, getting a wheelchair was liberating. Prior to having my own electric power chair, I felt like a potted plant. I could only move when someone pushed the wheelchair that I was placed in because my arms were too weak to push the wheels. While I worked intensively to be able to walk on my own, I realized after twelve weeks that it was unsafe, painful, and not practical, because I was so slow. Having an electric wheelchair was not a sign of disability but, rather, an opportunity to move by myself and go where I wanted to go.

Type of Wheelchair	Advantages	Disadvantqges
Manual Wheelchairs	• Lightweight • Greater reliability • Easier to transport • Less expensive • Provides exercise • Easier to overcome accessibility problems	Self-Propulsion: • Possible secondary complications after long-term use such as sore shoulders, wrists, and elbows • Requires physical effort to be mobile
Scooter Wheelchairs	• Aesthetics—does not look like a wheelchair. • Increases mobility range without increased exertion • Swivel seat may allow • for easier transfers in and out of the seat	• More complicated to transport in a car than a manual chair • Needs charging • Less flexible modifications to meet changing physical conditions than a power chair
Power Wheelchairs	• Greatest mobility range with least exertion • Easier to modify over time, if needed • Available power seating options (i.e., tilt and/or recline)	• More expensive • More difficult to transport • Less reliable than manual wheelchairs.

Table 3: Wheelchair comparisons

Choosing the right wheelchair (Table 3): Your health care team will be closely involved when it's time for you to choose a wheelchair, but being aware of the major issues will help you figure out what you need to address before you get into the specifics of choosing one. Depending on which wheelchair you choose, you may have to buy a new car or van to accommodate it. You'll need to ask:

• Who will you purchase it from, and how qualified and responsive is the company's repair staff?

• What is the reliability of your wheelchair and its brand, and how available are parts?

• How much will it cost? How much of the cost will your insurance company cover?

• How easy is it to push or drive?

Manual wheelchairs: Manual wheelchairs are designed to allow you to propel yourself or to allow a companion to push the chair for you. Self-propelled manual wheelchairs are equipped with large wheels; the rider self-propels using both arms to push the hand rims, and in some situations, both legs, or one arm and one leg. Self-propelled folding chairs are the most common design, because they are lightweight, easy to transport in a car, and often small enough to fit in the overhead bin of an airplane. A disadvantage of these chairs is that most do not have a cushion for pressure relief. You must raise yourself off the chair every few minutes to avoid pressure ulcers. This constant lifting can be hard on the shoulders and contribute to shoulder problems over time.

You may choose to add suspension systems to your chair, which smooths the ride considerably. The cost for better ride quality is the weight of the chair (the shock absorbers add a few pounds) and price (it's higher). There are self-propelled chairs that use a lever to push the wheels, which may be more ergonomic than the standard hand-rim push chairs. The most recent advance is the power-assisted self-propelled wheelchair. There are two types:

1. Power-assisted wheels. These wheelchairs are equipped with a larger wheel in which the hub has a battery and motor that increases the efficiency of manual propulsion while reducing the effort that the rider must exert on the wheels. These hybrid wheelchairs are more easily transported than electric power chairs because they weigh much less (40 to 75 pounds versus 200 to 400 pounds), and the wheels can be easily removed so it can be placed into a car trunk. The only downside is that the chairs are expensive ($5,000 to $8,000).

2. Models in which a small third wheel, which contains an electric motor, is attached to the frame and propels the wheelchair, while you are using the rim to push (Figure 30). The advantage over power-assisted chairs is primarily in weight and flexibility, since the third wheel can easily be added or detached.

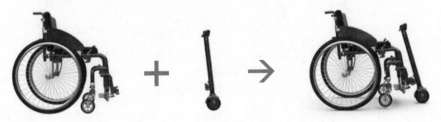

Figure 30. Attached motor assisted manual wheelchair

If you have impaired triceps function or any kind of shoulder problem, power-assisted chairs increase the distance and speed you can travel. Most important, they dramatically decrease damage to the shoulder's rotator cuff. Future advances in battery technology should improve performance, decrease weight, and lower costs.

Scooters: Scooters provide power mobility and have the advantage of not looking like a wheelchair. If you're feeling self-conscious about using a wheelchair or are limited by your endurance, a scooter may be right for you. If you've experienced difficulty walking, a scooter enables you to move faster and cover greater distances. Scooters are also relatively low in cost, lightweight, easily transported, and easy to get on and off, because the chair swivels. There are, however, a number of disadvantages that include a long turning radius, lack of stability on uneven surfaces (such as outdoors), and no ability to change seating options or cushions. They also require good upper body control, including arm and hand strength. If your physical performance declines, you may not be able to use a scooter because they have few functional adjustments.

Power electric wheelchairs: The most expensive and complex type of wheelchair has two major components: the power base (which contains the motors, wheels, batteries, and control module) and the seating component. The most obvious difference in power bases is the position of the drive wheel. Power wheelchair manufacturers offer three types of "drives": rear-wheel, mid-wheel, and front-wheel drive. The placement of the drive wheel has a significant impact on how the chair moves. Each method has its advantages and disadvantages in both indoor and outdoor driving conditions. Once you drive a power chair, you'll know which drive position is best for you, because it will require the least effort to go in a straight line and be the easiest to maneuver. It's also important to consider the battery. Choose a chair with gel or dry-cell batteries as opposed to liquid ones, which can spill corrosive lead acid. Gel and dry-cell batteries are lighter, maintenance-free, and approved for airline travel.

The seat consists of two components: 1) the seat cushion, and 2) a motor that enables multiple positions for the footrests and the backrests, as well as tilting the entire chair to optimize your comfort and posture, and provide pressure relief.

1. **Seat cushions:** To minimize the risk of pressure ulcers, you should consider special seat cushions. Similar to beds, there are several types of seat cushion material: foam, air, gel, and dynamic or hybrid. The right cushion should provide comfort, correct positioning, and prevent pressure ulcers. To choose a cushion that meets these requirements, ask your therapists and doctors for advice, then try out the cushion for twelve to eighteen hours to ensure that it's comfortable for you. Different cushions will distribute your weight more or less effectively. To help you choose the right cushion, you will likely use force sensing array (FSA) pressure mapping, which measures the interface pressure, the force per unit area (mm-Hg per square inch) between the body and the cushion. This is done by placing a thin rubber mat containing hundreds of pressure sensors on top of your cushion. When you sit on the mat, a technician records the maximum FSA under bony parts of your body as you assume different positions in the chair. The goal is to maintain peak FSA below 20mm-Hg per inch.

Among cushion materials, foam is the least expensive, is lightweight, and doesn't leak or lose air. It's not very durable, though, and does not provide pressure relief as effectively as other materials. Air cushions, such as the ROHO model, look like egg cartons with large black eggs arranged in rows, usually four to six rows per panel. Each panel can be inflated to its own pressure, allowing you excellent pressure relief (better than foam). They are also lightweight and allow the cushion to be adjusted to provide the best pressure relief for you individually. But they can leak (you need to check the inflation frequently), and they require adjustment when you change altitude. Gel cushions provide pressure relief and shear control equivalent to air cushions. Gel cushions weigh more, but you won't need to check their air pressure routinely, and they don't leak. I chose the Jay-2 cushion, which is a low-viscosity gel cushion, because of its excellent shock absorption (bumps make my shoulders hurt), good support (my trunk control was poor), and good pressure relief. Dynamic cushions, such as the Aquila, use a pump that alternates pressure throughout the cushion over time. While the integrated pump is theoretically better than other systems, many people find it impractical because it's expensive and noisy, requires batteries, and takes up space. For a list of available cushions and seating systems, check out the United

Spinal Association Disability Products & Services Directory, which has the greatest variety and most up-to-date information on disability products for everyone with ANI (more in the Resources on page 283).

2. **Power seating positions:** More expensive chairs allow you to adjust the seating positions. You can position them to tilt, recline, and elevate; the footrests are adjustable, and these chairs even enable you to stand. Tilting and reclining can help with pressure relief. Reclining changes the angle of your back so that true pressure relief is minimal, although it may be comfortable for rest and sleep. Tilting transfers weight to your back and off the bones of your pelvis, providing excellent pressure relief. Elevation not only enables you to reach objects on higher shelves but allows you to speak face-to-face with people who are standing, which is particularly nice in social situations. It can be difficult to carry on a conversation in a large, noisy room when you're seated two feet below everyone else, so being able to elevate the chair enhances your ability to have a conversation. It also makes it easier for people to see you and find you.

There are many important factors to keep in mind when choosing the chair itself, but it's also important to evaluate the chair in the places where you spend the most time: your home, your community, and your workplace.

Home: How accessible is your home? How easy is it to navigate inside your home? What is the width of the chair; will it fit through your doorways? How easy are transfers from the chair to the bed or couch? Can you adjust the height of the chair so that you can use a transfer board to get in and out of bed? How well does it fit in your kitchen and under your kitchen table? How maneuverable is it around your furniture? Does it bunch up or rip your rugs or carpeting?

Community: How will you get around in your community? How easy is it to get the wheelchair in and out of your van or car? If you can afford a van and have a power chair, you can lock it down with straps anchored in the floor, or use a floor locking mechanism that holds on to a pin installed in your van. If you have a car, you'll probably need to transfer from your wheelchair into the driver's seat. Depending on your strength, you may need a transfer board to get from chair to seat. Then, you should put your manual wheelchair in a location that enables you to retrieve it easily. If you plan to use your chair as your primary way to get around in your community, what is the terrain in your neighborhood: hilly or flat? Are there sidewalks, and what condition are they in? If there aren't any sidewalks, you will need emergency flashers to make yourself visible on the road, or you will have to find alternative routes. Are you planning to go out at night? If so, you will need headlights. Are you planning to go off-road onto trails, grass, or gravel? If so, you will need wider tires and more torque, as well as a more stable platform. What accessories will you need to function in your community? How will you carry your money and wallet, pills and water, phone and computer? You may consider using a backpack that attaches to the back of the chair, or a small bag that attaches under the front. Make sure your chair has places to attach these bags.

Work: How will you get to and into your workplace? Once inside, how will you get around? Will your desk accommodate your wheelchair? Will you need accessories for the chair during group meetings? Consider your workplace's unique circumstances as you select a wheelchair. And be sure to meet with someone in the human resources department to review your new needs and how they can be addressed. The Americans with Disabilities Act (ADA) outlines the necessary steps that the employer must perform for a qualified disabled individual, though the accommodations must be reasonable and cannot impose excessive hardship on the employer.

Walking—adaptive devices

Orthoses and braces: Orthoses control, guide, and limit an extremity or joint to improve function necessary for walking, reaching and grasping, and other specific movements. They also may reduce weight-bearing to protect a paralyzed or weak muscle. A lower-limb orthosis can improve walking by controlling the range of motion, stabilizing joints to prevent injury and maintain proper limb orientation, and reducing pain by transferring weight from a weak to a strong muscle group. If your injury has caused damage to your lower leg function, you may use an ankle-foot orthosis (AFO) to support the ankle and allow the foot to clear the ground during the swing phase of walking. If you have a more serious injury, you may require a knee-ankle-foot orthosis (KAFO) that allows you to stabilize the knee and ankle. While it's hard work, people using KAFOs, even those with no hip flexion, can take steps by swinging their legs while supported by forearm crutches.

Braces: Braces are used to provide additional support for a weakened joint or muscle. The most common is the knee brace, which reduces the risk of hyperextension and increases agility and strength of the knee. I use one for walking and riding my tricycle; it prevents my knee from wobbling, which can damage my knee joint and injure my thigh muscles (quadriceps sprain). The brace also decreases stress on the ligaments that maintain knee stability. Athletes, particularly football players, often use braces to prevent ligament tears, especially to the ACL and medial tendons.

Canes and walking sticks: You may need to use a cane if you have weakness on one side of your body. To support your weaker side, the cane is held in the hand of your *stronger* side as you walk. When selecting a cane, ensure it is the proper length for you; when your arm hangs by your side, the top of the cane should align with your wrist.

Walking sticks are useful if you have impaired balance due to damage to the parts of the brain that control your equilibrium and balance (e.g., the cerebellum, the motor and sensory portions of the cortex, and the vision center in the occipital lobe). Imbalance is usually due to loss of sensation, especially proprioception, the sense that tells your brain where your limbs are in space. Walking sticks usually contain a spring mechanism to help absorb shock, which is particularly useful when going downhill. You may find that you like to use walking sticks in both hands for ease of balance.

Crutches: If you need to use crutches to recover from injuries to your legs, you will have a choice of two basic types: those that sit under your arm or those that are cuffed to your forearm. Your therapy team will help you decide which style is best for you. Either way, a proper fit is critical, since ill-fitting crutches can cause blisters on your hands and underarms as well as nerve damage to the brachial plexus that travels through your armpit, which could cause you to stumble and fall.

Walkers: Walkers come in many designs based on their complexity and speed (Figure 31). Choose a walker based on your balance, leg and arm strength, and endurance.

- Standard walker: This has four nonskid, rubber-tipped legs that provide stability (Figure 31A). You must pick it up to move, which allows people with limited balance to walk over uneven surfaces.

- Front-wheeled walker: This design is good if you need some, but not constant, weight-bearing help. It has a hard plastic cup called a glide on the rear legs to enable you to stop and rest, and also provides more control while walking (Figure 31B). If you have weak triceps and shoulder muscles, you can raise the height so that you can rest your forearms on special arm pads. This is called a platform walker, which is what I use (Figure 32).

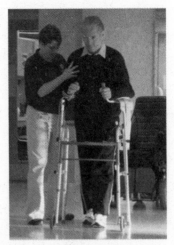

Figure 32. Platform walker

- Four-wheel walker: This type is best for people who don't need to lean on the walker for balance. With four wheels, it has the advantage of being able to move faster than two-wheeled walkers, and it can be equipped with a brake (Figure 31C).

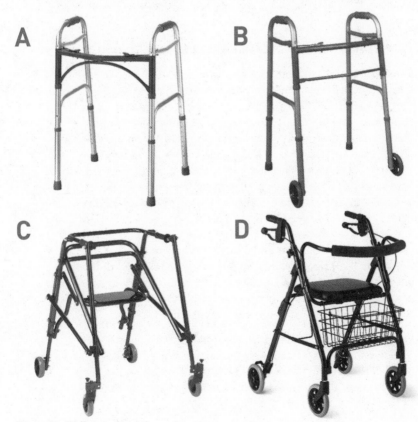

Figure 31. Walkers

- Rollator or rolling walker: These consist of a frame with four large wheels, handlebars, and a built-in seat, which allows you to stop and rest when needed (Figure 31D). They frequently have hand brakes to control speed. Rolling walkers are most commonly used for walking longer distances, and for activities such as grocery shopping and taking a walk. They can be customized to accommodate a bag or basket.

Preventing Falls

Falls are one of the most common reasons people are readmitted to the hospital. Usually, the fall is caused by an ANI-related symptom, such as poor vision, dizziness, weakness on one side, lack of sensation, spasticity, or poor balance; and an environmental hazard, such as a slippery floor, steep or poorly lighted stairs with insufficient handrails, and/or tight spaces. Add in a difficult movement like getting out of bed, and you have a recipe for a fall.

New Technologies: Exoskeletons and Exosuits

Exoskeletons: Exoskeletons are battery-powered mechanical leg braces that use small motors at the joints to assist in walking (Figure 29; page 186). The ReWalk Personal System (Figure 29A; page 186) combines a brace support for legs and abdomen, a computer-based control system, and motion sensors. Videos on the ReWalk website show paraplegics standing and walking independently, and *very* excited to be moving on their own. But exoskeletons are very expensive ($75,000 to $125,000), making them inaccessible to most people. They are also slow (allowing walking at the speed of 1 or 2 miles per hour versus 2 to 5 miles per hour in a manual or power chair), and require ten to twenty minutes to put on and take off. To use them, you must also have near-normal upper body strength and endurance. When you transition from a hospital setting to rehabilitation or home, use of an exoskeleton will require a well-trained and dedicated caregiver. For these reasons, I don't believe that exoskeleton technology will replace the wheelchair anytime soon.

Exosuits: Exosuits are designed for stroke patients who have leg weakness greater than arm weakness on one side. The ReWalk device is called ReStore (Figure 29B; page 186). It consists of a powered ankle and foot device that helps you plant your foot and lift it up so that you can walk faster and more evenly.

Walking devices such as canes, crutches, and walkers provide balance and control to prevent falls. To assist you as you get out of bed and go from sitting to standing, you can use a handrail that has been securely inserted under your mattress or a more sophisticated bar, such as the ones found on hospital beds. To make it easier to get up from a chair, you can use an electric reclining chair that slowly pushes you forward.

The bathroom is a particularly dangerous place because of slippery floors and tight spaces. Handrails and grab bars in places where you need support are inexpensive solutions. If standing in the shower is difficult, you may need a shower seat that folds down from the wall or a shower chair that rolls into the shower. Going up and down stairs may be risky; you can have handrails and nonslip stair-tread coverings installed. If you are too weak to climb stairs, there are motorized seats that carry you up and down. Whatever your personal and environmental risks for fall, you should purchase a fall detection monitoring device and alarm. Older models require you to press a call button that activates a telephone call for emergency help. Newer models have an accelerometer and GPS that can automatically detect when and where you have fallen and send out that information immediately.

Sports

You will probably be surprised to learn how many sports can be played with adaptive devices. Let's start with wheelchair sports. These include basketball, billiards, bowling, golf, rugby, tennis, and wheelchair racing. For me, the most exciting adaptive sport to watch is racing because it has been the sport where the most unique and sophisticated adaptations have occurred. The racing wheelchair has three wheels: a small one in front and two large ones, as on a normal wheelchair, where the person sits. The adaptations include wind-tunnel aerodynamic designs and use of carbon fiber frames and solid disc wheels. The official marathon world record is 1:20:14 (forty minutes faster than the running marathon record!). An important concept is that you can take a piece of sporting equipment for nondisabled people and adapt it to your own specific needs. Some examples are cycling, horseback riding, and skiing (water and snow). I use a recumbent tricycle (Figure 33) that has pedals in the front, which allows me to see my legs moving so that I can keep them straight; because I cannot feel them, I wouldn't know if I was pedaling properly otherwise.

In addition, I had the controls for the brakes and gears shifted to my left hand, because I could not use them with my weak right hand.

Standing frames

Standing has many physical benefits: It helps prevent pressure ulcers, improves circulation, increases range of motion, and reduces spasms and contractions. Studies have shown that people who stand for thirty minutes or more each day have a better quality of life, fewer pressure ulcers and bladder infections, increased bone density, and better bowel function than those who don't stand at all. To increase your standing time, you may want to acquire a standing frame (Figure 22; page 150). My physiatrist recommended that I get one to maintain bone density in my hips and legs. If you have difficulty standing independently for more than thirty minutes at a time, you may benefit from a standing frame. It's best to stand every day, starting with five minutes and working up to sixty minutes. I use mine every day, and I've noticed improvements in my circulation and gastrointestinal health. Your health care team will guide you on how and when you should use a standing frame.

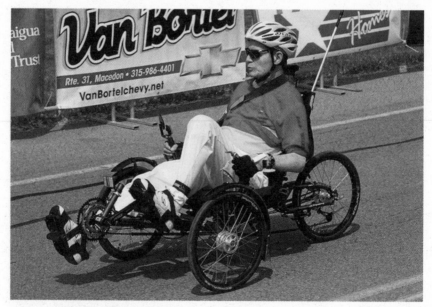

Figure 33. Three-wheeled recumbent tricycle

Aids for Daily Living

Bathing: After ANI, there are important reasons for daily showers beyond getting clean. Showers provide opportunities for a thorough skin check (ask your partner or aide to check the parts of your body you can't see). Look for abrasions, cuts, bruises, or developing pressure ulcers, and be sure to deal with them immediately, if found. If you have paralysis or weakened limbs, you may find showers to be easier than baths, because getting out of a bathtub can be a risky maneuver.

Your ability to bathe yourself is determined largely by the range of motion of your arms and dexterity of your hands. If you have limited use of your arms, you'll need a shower chair and assistance taking a shower. Even if you can transfer to a shower seat yourself or stand in the shower by holding on to grab bars, it's still helpful to have someone nearby in case you need help. If you are able, you may want to consider building a roll-in shower, which makes entering and exiting the shower easier and safer—with or without a wheelchair—and eliminates a trip hazard.

Toileting: Having a bowel movement poses significant logistical problems for many people. If you have decreased mobility, especially decreased standing and walking, you're at risk for constipation. The motility of your bowels that is necessary to propel stool is decreased in people with dysfunction of the autonomic nervous system, which is common in SCI above T6, and in stroke and TBI patients with brain damage (especially to the insular cortex).

You'll likely need several adaptive devices for the bathroom, including a shower commode-chair that fits over the 14-inch (35 cm) standard-height toilet with more than 4 inches (10 cm) of room between the seat and the toilet rim. This allows you to reach your anus to perform digital stimulation (using your finger to push against your anus and rectum, causing a reflex action of your colon muscles and pushing the stool out), if necessary. You'll also need a flushing mechanism that is easy to reach and activate, a suppository inserter, and a digital stimulation device if you cannot reach your anus with your fingers.

Grooming and hygiene: Grooming requires adaptation of existing devices. After my injury, I switched from a razor blade to an electric razor for shaving, purchased a hairbrush with an extra-long handle, and bought an ultrasonic toothbrush so that I don't need to move my hand to brush my teeth.

I also increased the size of the ultrasonic toothbrush handle by wrapping it with Dycem Non-Slip material, to make it sticky and easy to hold. To floss my teeth, I switched from the usual string to portable hand-held flossers called Plackers. There are many other grooming tasks that may require assistance if you don't have good hand and arm function (e.g., makeup; shaving armpits and legs; washing, drying, and styling hair).

Clothing: You may have to alter your wardrobe to match your abilities and avoid your limitations. The two major obstacles to dressing yourself are zippers and buttons. The solutions are Velcro and self-threading zippers that snap together with magnets. You can also find clothing online that's tailored for people with paralysis. It's frequently called accessible and inclusive fashion (see the Resources on page 283). If you have a good local tailor, it may be less expensive to have them modify your current clothing. For example, I had an extra-long overcoat altered into a cape. The cape has a back that is cut open halfway up so that it doesn't bunch when I sit down in the wheelchair; I also had the side panels removed but kept the pockets, and I had a slit made to put my arms through. A zipper with a big ring replaced the buttons, and the buttons were reattached with Velcro backing, so that the right and left sides stay buttoned over the zipper. The cape is easy to put on and take off, comfortable to wear, and covers my legs, providing extra warmth and protection.

Shoes: Velcro closures make it easy to put on and take off your shoes, and a low back makes a shoe easy to step into. Soft materials on the shoe itself, such as cotton, wool, or flexible leather (which can be found in lightweight shoes and sneakers), can help prevent pressure ulcers. The sole should not be leather, which can be slippery, but rather a synthetic material that provides better traction for transfers and repositioning if you use a wheelchair.

Eating: Eating independently is an important part of building self-esteem and increasing quality of life after your injury. But frequently, the strength, range of motion, and fine-motor control you need to use standard utensils is lacking. Fortunately, there are excellent assistive devices for eating. If you have sufficient biceps and deltoid strength, you may be able to use a mobile arm support (MAS) or balanced forearm orthosis (BFO) to help with eating, grooming, and hygiene (Figure 34). As you regain strength and endurance, you may not need to continue using the MAS. If you're too weak or unsteady to hold a glass, you might need a straw to drink from a cup. A next step would be to use a water bottle with a straw that goes to the bottom so you can drink without having to turn the bottle upside down.

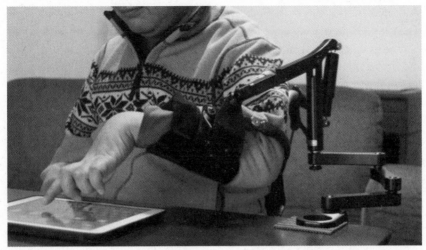

Figure 34. Balanced forearm orthosis (BFO)

If you have limited hand and finger strength, a common adaptive device for eating is the universal cuff, which accepts many utensils with handles (Figure 35). You also may choose to use Dycem (to help hold your dishes in place) and a plate guard (to prevent you from pushing your food off the plate). For many months, I used a fork with a universal cuff and then a Dining with Dignity fork (Figure 36) to push my food against the plate guard to get it to stay on the fork. These were very helpful for developing the ability to feed myself independently.

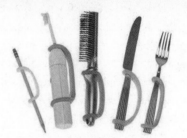

Figure 35. Universal cuffs for handheld items

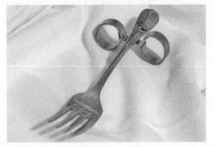

Figure 36. Dining with Dignity fork

Holding and carrying: If you have weak arms or limited hand function, you may have trouble holding things like books, phones, and tablets. One of my favorite solutions is the gooseneck tablet holder, which can be mounted to any flat surface, including your chair, bed, or desk. One of the difficulties of living in a wheelchair is that it's hard to carry things with you, since you need your hands to push the wheel rims or drive your electric power chair. Fortunately, there are lots of solutions for carrying items, such as a backpack. The advantage of a backpack is that the storage volume is quite large and can be well organized, but since it's placed on the back of your chair, you may not be able to reach it easily. If you use a manual wheelchair, you can use a small bag attached under the seat to hold a few items, such as your wallet, phone, and snacks. I like using a tray that rests on my knees because I can see my items—phone, tablet, papers, and books—in front of me. It's also a good surface for eating; I put Dycem on the tray or rubber coasters to hold a plate and cup.

Transfer devices: Most people with paralysis develop the ability to perform a sit-pivot transfer or use a transfer board. If you have strong arms, you can use them to push yourself up and over. If you have strong legs, you can do a sit-to-stand quadriceps push and then sideways rotation. If you're too weak to do a sit-pivot transfer, there are several types of devices you can use to transfer between surfaces of similar heights (e.g., bed to chair), and surfaces of different heights (e.g., chair to exam table). Many people use a sliding or transfer board (slick wood or plastic) to facilitate transfers, but these can only help when the surfaces are of similar heights, or the surface you're transferring to is lower. But be aware that sliding causes more shear force on your pelvis than a sit-pivot transfer and therefore predisposes you to pressure ulcers. You can reduce the shear force by making sure the surface of the board has very little friction, and by wearing slick pants, such as those made from polyester or acrylic material (blue jeans are the absolute worst for transferring!). If you don't have enough core strength to safely perform a sit-pivot or sliding-board transfer, you can use a mechanical lift, such as the Hoyer lift (Figure 37). A comfortable sling is placed under your bottom and is then attached securely to an arm that extends to move you in the desired direction.

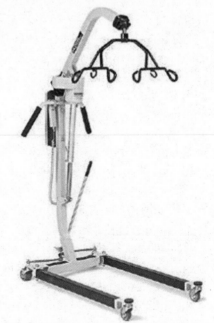

Figure 37. Hoyer lift

Wearables: These small devices (including smart watches) that are worn on your body can measure calories expended by monitoring heart rate and activity (number of steps, distance traveled by walking or in a manual wheelchair). It's important to understand your energy expenditure so you can maintain the right level of exercise. Newer devices can measure your blood pressure, breathing rate, and blood oxygen levels, providing real-time information on your health.

How to Pay for Adaptive Devices and Assistive Technology

Your health insurance should pay for some or all of the assistive devices you need. But if it doesn't, a great place to start looking for help is the Assistive Technology Industry Association, which offers a free Funding Resources Guide. They also provide helpful information on choosing devices.

Some of the other methods of funding include:

- school systems (if you are a student) that distribute specialized materials as well as assistive technology specified in an Individual Education Plan (IEP) or a 504 plan

- government programs (Social Security, Veterans Benefits Administration, or state Medicaid agencies) that pay for assistive technology if a doctor prescribes it as a medically necessary device

- private health insurance companies, which pay for assistive technology if a doctor prescribes it as a necessary medical or rehabilitative device

- rehabilitation and job-training programs, funded by government or private agencies, which may pay for assistive technology and employment training to help people get jobs

- employers that pay for assistive technology as a reasonable accommodation to enable an employee to perform essential job tasks

- private foundations, charities, and civic organizations (see the Resources section on page 283 for a complete list)

Adaptive devices and assistive technology are expanding dramatically as the "Internet of Things" becomes more and more a part of daily life. Devices that control your environment, your security, and your food preparation are already transforming your home, and will continue to do so.

Everything You Need to Know

Adaptive devices and assistive technology will greatly enhance your quality of life. Begin discussing and researching your options as soon after your injury as possible, while you are still in the hospital. Involve members of your household in the process. Keep a notebook with notes on device options, manufacturer brochures, prescriptions from your doctor, funding options, and so on.

As you progress in outpatient rehabilitation, your needs may change. Keep your physician informed so that if your health insurance company requires a prescription for a new device, one will be available.

Some assistive devices are inexpensive and for short-term use; others are expensive and meant to be useful for years. Be sure to investigate your options thoroughly so that you can make the choices that are best for you. Whenever possible, ask your rehabilitation program if you can try high-ticket items for a week. Many of them have donated chairs and beds that you can test.

Don't let cost deter you from purchasing the best devices and AT for you; investigate the community, state, regional, and national organizations that exist to provide funds that help.

16

Get Out!

Making Your Home, Vehicles, and Workplace
Accessible for a Wheelchair

THE HOUSE MY WIFE and I lived in prior to my injury was a lovely English Tudor-style home built in 1929. A flight of steps led to the front door, and the primary bedroom and bath were on the second floor. There were lots of doorways and thresholds and corners to turn as you went from room to room. After my accident, we discussed remodeling plans with three different contractors, but it soon became apparent that the cost to make the house accessible—to meet my new needs—would be prohibitive. Fortunately, we found a townhouse that had everything I needed. Saying goodbye to our old house and all the happy memories we made there was difficult. But staying was not an option we could afford. The relative ease of living in the townhouse made the transition easier, which helped me focus on rehabilitation and my goal of returning to work as soon as possible.

Depending on your mobility and needs, it is quite likely that you'll need to make some modifications, especially if you're going to use a wheelchair. The three most important areas to optimize for functionality and mobility are: 1) your home (entrance and doorways, bathroom, bedroom, and kitchen); 2) your transportation (a van or a modified car); and 3) your workplace (accessible). The changes that will matter most to you are safety and return on investment—spending money on things that will have the biggest impact on your quality of life. Your occupational therapist, social worker, and members of your support group can provide you with advice on how best to navigate this new situation.

Your Home

The first major decision in making your home accessible is determining if it's possible and how much it will cost. The second is determining how much renovation you really need. Are you a committed chef who will need lower countertops and special appliances, like ovens with shorter depths, to enable you to reach in and pull out pans without burning yourself? Do you really need an accessible hot tub in your bathroom? For most of us, the answer is no. The three most important design features in your home will be an accessible bathroom (frequently with a roll-in shower for a shower commode chair), a first-floor bedroom and bathroom, and no carpeting and few rugs, if you are using a wheelchair or a cane. Having hardwood floors makes it easier to push your wheelchair or walk with crutches, a cane, or a walker. Even if you reach a point where you don't need assistive devices, you may consider removing wall-to-wall carpeting and area rugs, as they can be trip hazards.

Before you make any renovations, try to visit the homes of people with disabilities similar to yours; ask your friends and support group members to put you in touch with people who have similar needs to learn about their modifications. Check out home designs online. Talk to your physical and occupational therapists, and have them visit your house to see the space. Contact your chamber of commerce for a list of local builders with experience in accessible renovations. Many contractors follow the design/build method, which means their plans only need sign-off from an engineer (and not an architect) to obtain a building permit. If you decide to hire an architect, be sure to hire one with expertise in accessible living and ask to see at least three previous projects.

Entrance and doorways: While newer homes, especially ranch-style houses, may be readily accessible, many older homes have stairs to all entrance doors. All homes should be equipped with two accessible exits for emergencies, such as fire. If you live in an area with significant snowfall and have an attached garage, you'll want a ramp installed from the garage into the house. Every state has its own building codes, but a typical ramp would be at least 3 feet (91 cm) wide, with a pitch of less than 12 inches (30 cm) length for every 1 inch (2.5 cm) in rise, and with a railing that is at least 32 inches (81 cm) high. If the ramp has to change direction, there should be a 5-foot-by-5-foot (1.5 x 1.5 m) platform at that intersection. Ramps can be made of wood, wood-plastic composites, or metal (usually aluminum), and should have a nonskid material covering the surface. Wood (pressure-treated lumber or durable wood, like teak) is used most frequently because it is the least expensive material. Engineered wood-plastic composites are becoming more popular as their prices approach that of wood. They have several advantages over wood ramps: no warping, splitting, or splintering, and no need for repainting or re-staining. Lightweight aluminum, though most expensive, is also a good material, especially if the ramp needs to be relocated, because it's the easiest to disassemble and move.

For doorways, a minimum width of 32 inches (81 cm) is recommended to enable easy passage in a wheelchair. If the doorway is too narrow (many older homes have 30-inch/76 cm wide doorways), you are likely to scrape your fingers, hands, and arms as you pass through. You are also likely to scratch the paint on the doorway, and you may damage your wheelchair's arm supports. To widen your doorways, you can remove the doors or install pocket doors that slide into the wall. If you have standard doors in your home, you may consider changing the doorknobs. Opening a standard door with a doorknob requires significant reach and grasp capabilities, which may be beyond your ability. Replace your doorknobs with a mechanism that is easy to grasp with one hand and doesn't require much strength to move, like a lever. To modify existing doorknobs, attach a rubber snap-on lever that fits over them. A remote-controlled door opener, like those commonly used for garage doors, is another good solution. Thresholds should be no higher than ¾ inch (2 cm) in height. If your thresholds are higher, you may need to install a small wooden or aluminum ramp to make it easier to roll over them.

Bathroom: The bathroom, of all the rooms in the home, usually requires the most remodeling. A standard bathtub and shower won't work if you have problems with strength, coordination, balance, and vision. If you're able to transfer from your wheelchair independently, your existing shower may work, as long as it isn't part of a bathtub and the entrance is close to a wall and wide enough so that you can transfer onto a bench. In most cases, you will need to add a shower chair or bench, grab bars, and a shower wand so you can shower on your own. If you're unable to transfer independently, you will need to transfer from your bed or your wheelchair onto a special-ized shower chair that you or an aide can roll into the shower.

If you use a wheelchair, you will likely need to modify your bathroom sink; if not, you should be OK with a standard sink and a grab bar. To control the water temperature and flow, a single-handle faucet is the best choice. The sink should measure about 30 inches (75 cm) wide, 19 inches (50 cm) front to back, and less than 6.5 inches (16.5 cm) deep. It should be mounted to the wall, 27 to 32 inches (68–81 cm) high, *without* a cabinet underneath so that you can roll up to it in your wheelchair, with adequate space below the sink to accommodate your knees. Hang mirrors over the sink (and other places in the house) so that you can see yourself from both a seated and standing position.

The toilet should be standard height (14–18 inches/35–45 cm from the floor to rim) with a minimum of 18 inches (45 cm) of space on both sides of the bowl. You may need to install a grab bar on one or both sides of the toilet, if it's in an alcove. Maintaining the bathroom at a warm temperature (70–78°F/21–25°C) is critical and can best be achieved with infrared lights or heat lamps, which are faster and more efficient (and less expensive) than a heated floor.

Kitchen: How much time do you spend in the kitchen? While some people will want a customized kitchen they can cook in, for many of us, being able to reach into the fridge and put a prepared meal in the microwave is sufficient for a typical meal. This can be accomplished by having a drawer refrigerator or a side-by-side refrigerator in which you keep your most commonly used items on the lower shelves if you are in a wheelchair, or at chest level if you are standing with a walker or cane. You can place a microwave on a table or countertop at a height of 27 to 32 inches (68–81 cm) for easy access. Ovens and dishwashers can be challenging due to their pull-down doors, which can make putting items in and taking them out quite difficult, but there are few commercially available solutions. I use a large countertop convection toaster oven (16 x 20 x 11 inches/40 x 50 x 28 cm) that can accommodate six slices of toast, a whole roast chicken, a personal pan pizza, and other large items. It has a handle so I can easily open and close it, and it's shallow, so I can easily reach in and out.

Bedroom: The most important features of a bedroom are easy access to the bathroom and sufficient space around the bed to maneuver a wheelchair easily, especially for transfer to the bed. There should be a minimum of 3 feet (1 m) on your side of the bed for transfers, and 4 feet (1.2 m) at the end of the bed for turning.

Other features you may wish to consider include a bed that is the same height as your wheelchair seat; a light switch, telephone, and clock that are easily accessible at the bedside; drawers that you can open with one hand; and storage for items that you use frequently, such as braces, prostheses, bedclothes, gloves, alcohol wipes, urine bags, and other medical supplies. Don't use electric blankets, because you could quickly develop a burn without feeling it.

Other modifications: If you'll be using a wheelchair, walker, cane, or crutches, you'll have difficulty maneuvering on plush carpeting. The Americans with Disabilities Act Standards for Accessible Design recommends that carpet pile should be no more than ½ inch (1 cm) thick. Throw rugs can move or bunch up under wheelchairs equipped with a docking pin (for securing the chair in a van), and they present a trip hazard if you're on crutches.

You may also need to make modifications to your electrical appliances. If you are remodeling your home, new electrical outlets should be placed at least 15 inches (38 cm) above the floor, and light switches and thermostats should be no higher than 48 inches (122 cm) above the floor. If your light switches and electrical outlets are not accessible to you, you can use a smart plug that works with your home automation systems (Amazon Echo, Google Nest, or Apple HomeKit) to allow you to control lights or other electrical devices without touching them.

As the baby boomer population ages, builders and developers are creating new homes with single-floor living, walk-in showers with no thresholds, built-in shower seats, "comfort height" toilets, grab bars, and open floor plans that only have doors to bedrooms and bathrooms. New construction often includes pocket doors for bedrooms and bathrooms, rather than hinged doors. This trend is to your advantage if you decide your best option is to move to another house.

Transportation

Driving with a disability often means relearning how to drive. The rules of the road don't change, but the controls do. Depending on your needs, an adapted vehicle (a van or modified car) may include something as simple as a spinner knob attached to the steering wheel for one-handed steering, if one upper limb is much weaker than the other. More complex devices include hand controls for braking and accelerating mounted on the steering wheel. There are also power-assist devices to enable you to drive by essentially moving a joystick.

Choosing the right vehicle and controls: Once you're ready to drive, you should take a driver's education course again. Most communities offer driving lessons for people with disabilities. Don't be surprised if this process is difficult for you. Slowly braking on a downhill slope in a

5,000-pound van isn't easy! Driver's ed teachers who help people with disabilities will have hands-on experience and knowledge of what type of vehicle and special controls you will need. In my experience, it's wise to underestimate your abilities so that if you hurt yourself, get sick, or develop chronic musculoskeletal problems, you will still be able to drive your vehicle.

Once you've completed driver's ed, you should be able to answer the most important question: *Do I want to drive independently, or should I find someone to be my driver?* I found driving to be mentally and physically tiring, so I ultimately decided not to drive myself.

If you're living with paralysis, ask yourself what kind of vehicle is right for you and whether adapting a car you already own is possible. Will you be driving from a wheelchair, thus requiring a van, or can you transfer to the car seat of a smaller passenger car? If you can transfer into a car, you will be able to purchase a less expensive vehicle, and you'll have many more choices. If you choose to drive from your wheelchair, will you and your wheelchair fit in the vehicle? If you're on the taller side, you may have difficulty getting into a car without your head hitting the door frame or pressing against the ceiling while you drive.

So, make sure to **buy your wheelchair before you buy your vehicle.** Proper wheelchair size is also important, so that your knees fit under the steering wheel, and your arm position is comfortable, particularly if you'll be driving for more than an hour at a stretch. Can the vehicle accommodate hand controls or other needed equipment such as a ramp, a place to store your wheelchair (not likely with a convertible), and a mechanism to lock your chair?

Will a full-size van fit in your garage? Once the van is parked in your garage, is there room for you to get out safely, especially if you need a ramp?

Once you decide what type of car would best suit you, you'll need to figure out how to pay for it. This usually requires significant financial assistance. Start with your state's Department of Vocational Rehabilitation and if appropriate, the Department of Veterans Affairs. If you are fortunate, as I was, your employer may make a significant contribution as part of their employment policies regarding people with disabilities. Other sources include not-for-profit agencies that have grant programs for individuals with disabilities; workers' compensation, if you were injured while working; rebates from automobile manufacturers; and state waivers for sales tax, if your physician prescribes the vehicle as medically necessary.

In most cases, you'll need to modify your car or van to your specifications. The cost of modifying a vehicle varies greatly. A new vehicle modified with adaptive equipment can cost anywhere from $30,000 to $90,000. If you receive funds to cover the cost of your modified car or van, make sure you ask about what will be covered; get precise details. Then have the seller provide detailed written specifications for the vehicles that are approved by the funding agency.

There are many available options for cars and vans, depending on whether you plan to buy one new or used. If you can afford it, the best approach is to purchase a new vehicle from the manufacturer and have it sent directly to a nationally recognized company that specializes in modifications of vehicles, like BraunAbility or Amerivan. If you plan to adapt a used van or car, be careful; unlike most people, if your vehicle breaks down, it won't be easy to find a loaner car! Therefore, you should have the vehicle inspected by a competent mechanic before buying it. When seeking out auto body shops to do the modification, choose ones that have proven expertise. In my metropolitan area of 1 million people, there's only one auto shop that has enough expertise to install locking systems and repair broken ramps. The best shops, like the one I use, make sure that they get it right. Shops that lack experience or cut corners will deliver a subpar vehicle that is always in need of repair.

Once you've determined what the specifications for your van or car need to be, it's time to learn more from friends, online forums, and community groups. Ask your friends what they like about their cars or vans and what they would change if they could do it all over again. Then make sure that your driver's ed instructor, occupational therapist, and physical therapist agree with your selection of vehicle and controls.

Public transportation: Federal laws, such the Americans with Disabilities Act (ADA), require all transportation providers to accommodate wheelchairs. Many states have antidiscrimination laws that require companies to treat all customers equally. Several large US cities (e.g., Chicago, New York, and Washington, DC) have mandated that taxi companies maintain a certain number of wheelchair-accessible vans, and most cities have buses with lifts to enable them to transport people using wheelchairs or rolling walkers. With advance notice, some public bus and taxi companies will send a vehicle to you. Subways are usually wheelchair-accessible, but getting to them may be difficult. For example, in New York City, only one in four subway stops has elevators, so you may need to travel on the sidewalk for five to twenty blocks to get to your destination.

Trains are probably the most accessible form of transportation in the US. All stations have an accessible entrance to the train, such as a ramp or an elevator, and the trains all have wheelchair-accessible seating. But getting on and off the train can be difficult, because sometimes there are many people crowding the exit. It may also be difficult for the conductor and other employees to assist you. To ensure that you get to your destination safely, talk to an employee prior to your scheduled stop so that they can be nearby to help you get off. Air travel is much friendlier for people with disabilities—we'll discuss that in chapter 17.

Workplace

Companies with more than fifty employees are required to modify the workplace to make it accessible as mandated by the ADA (see below for modifications). But even smaller companies that are exempt from ADA rules are usually willing to accommodate disabled employees, and national organizations exist to help small businesses make their workplaces accessible. Companies are also supposed to accommodate acquired cognitive disabilities, as may occur with ANI, especially TBI. If this applies to you, you should have a formal neuropsychology exam performed and the results submitted to your employer.

Employer-mandated responsibilities: The ADA mandates accessibility in schools, workplaces, public spaces, and transportation, and increased awareness of the need for universal design principles that make indoor and outdoor spaces accessible to people with disabilities. Title I of the ADA prohibits private employers, state and local governments, employment agencies, and labor unions from discriminating against qualified people with disabilities when it comes to job applications, hiring, firing, promotion, pay scale, job training, and other conditions and privileges of employment. A qualified employee is simply someone who, with or without reasonable accommodation, can perform the essential functions of the job in question.

Making work accessible and comfortable: Reasonable accommodation is an adjustment to make the existing workspace accessible and usable by people with disabilities. These might include ramps for entrance and emergency exit, wider doorways, room to maneuver in your office, desk and computer in ergonomic positions, and an accessible bathroom. It also includes other accommodations such as changing work hours. I changed my starting time from 7:30 AM to 9:30 because it takes me two hours to get ready for work, compared to 20 minutes pre-injury. Depending on your abilities, you may need assistance throughout the day to help you work, use a bathroom, go to meetings, and translate (e.g., sign language, if you've lost your hearing or have aphasia).

Resources to prevent discrimination: While there's a legal responsibility for employers to make reasonable accommodations, things don't always go smoothly. The good news is that there are several federal and state laws that will support your efforts to work. The bad news is that after you initiate an action against your employer, you may face hostility because the process is time consuming, expensive, and distracting for all parties involved. If you feel you've been a victim of discrimination, the resources available to you include the United States Equal Employment Opportunity Commission (EEOC), the Disability and Business Technical Assistance Centers, the Fair Employment Practice Agency (FEPA), and the Ticket to Work and Work Incentives Improvement Act (programs within the Social Security Administration). The EEOC is usually the first resource to turn to, since all major employers will have someone in human resources who can work with you and the EEOC.

Everything You Need to Know

Involve your family and your therapy team to help you improve your access to all the things that contribute to your quality of life—at home, at work, and on the road. That discussion will include:

- your home and what needs to be done to it to accommodate your new needs

- your transportation needs and whether you should drive or enlist someone to drive you, as well as whether your car or van can be modified or will need to be replaced

- your workplace and what may need to be done to accommodate you before you return to work.

- a support group—one that meets in a physical location or online (Your fellow group members can guide your choices with their real-life experiences.)

17

When the World Beckons

The Good, Bad, and Worst of
Traveling in a Wheelchair

TRAVELED FREQUENTLY BEFORE MY injury, for both business and pleasure. I attended medical research conferences around the world, and my family and I enjoyed vacations on a regular basis. I didn't want to give that up just because I spend most of my day in a wheelchair. But I soon learned that traveling in a wheelchair was a much more challenging endeavor than I'd imagined. I didn't give up, and as a result, I can share with you everything I wish I'd known on those early trips.

While each form of transportation has its own set of challenges for a person in a wheelchair, these are the important issues to address for all types of travel:

- **Planning in advance is critical.** Whenever possible, work with a travel agent who has expertise in arranging trips for people with disabilities. You want to be sure that your accommodations, and any tours or excursions, are accessible. In terms of air travel, most large US airlines have specialty agents who can assist with disability travel. They are particularly helpful if any of your equipment is damaged while being transported.

- **Making your needs known to the staff is essential.** While traveling and at your destination, make sure that the crew and staff know about your limitations; inform them when you need special treatment or encounter a problem. Emergency preparedness lends peace of mind to you and your companions before and during the trip. That means acknowledging that big problems can happen, so use a credit card that includes medical transport by air if needed. In some situations, consider purchasing trip insurance, usually about 5 percent of the total cost of your trip. A travel agent will advise when purchasing insurance is a good idea.

Planning for Your Trip

There are three options for planning a travel experience. You can do it yourself (DIY), use a travel agent, or go on a tour. It's best to wait to try DIY until you've completed at least five trips, since there are many tasks—hotels, airlines, trip insurance, and ground transportation—that will require hours of online and telephone time. Even someone who was an experienced traveler before acquiring a disability faces potential obstacles to an enjoyable trip. That's why I recommend that you work with a travel agent who has experience in arranging trips for people with your particular needs or go on a tour that is designed for people with disabilities. A number of organizations, such as AAA Member Choice Vacations, AARP (formerly called the American Association for Retired Persons), and Costco, offer all-inclusive packages (airfare, transfers, hotel, food and drink, and tours). And, of course, you can talk to friends who use wheelchairs so that you can learn from their travel experiences. Planning means getting started *six months before your trip* whenever possible. The number of accessible places to stay is limited, and the details of excursions at your destination require extra time to plan as well.

Tours and cruises are the easiest trips to take. There are several companies that specialize in accessible tours, which you can find online or through a good travel agent. These groups are usually cost-effective compared to regular tours because there's a pooling of expenses—six couples can share the cost of renting a wheelchair lift van, for example. And the places where you stay during these tours usually have experienced staff to help. As I was writing this book, my wife and I found a ten-day tour on wheelchairtravel.org for ten to twelve people to Lisbon, Portugal, for $3,500 per person. That included hotels, meals, ground transportation—all major expenses except for airfare. The tour company does all the planning (museums, historic sites, tickets to cultural events, and so on), which saves an enormous amount of work.

Cruises are particularly well-suited for the wheelchair traveler. You stay in the same cabin (room) during your travels, while the ship sails from place to place. Recently, several cruise lines have begun to offer special excursion tours for wheelchair users. For example, Disney Cruise Line has forty-six accessible shore excursions in thirty-nine ports around the world, making cruise vacations more accessible than ever to people with disabilities. The excursions are led by professional tour guides and feature accessible accommodations. Specialized vehicles with wheelchair ramps or lifts are provided, and the tours follow step-free routes to ensure access for people with limited mobility.

Paying for Your Trip

Using a credit card for your travel expenses will enable you to obtain insurance at a low-cost or even as a benefit of the credit card. It will also facilitate resolving any disagreements with the travel partners involved in your vacation (such as airlines, ground transportation, car rentals, hotels, tours). For people with disabilities, the best choice is the card that offers the most comprehensive travel insurance, compensation for delayed or lost baggage, and medical coverage. Paying attention to details will make the difference between a great trip and a horrible one. If, suddenly, you're unable to take a trip because of an illness, a death in the family, or a natural disaster, you'd face a huge financial loss if you didn't have travel insurance. The right credit card can offer travel insurance for coverage when your travel doesn't go as planned. There are several websites that compare the travel benefits of different credit cards, such as NerdWallet and WalletHub—and you should also ask your frequent-flyer friends for advice. Because these benefits can and do change, you may want to call customer service to confirm what you find online. As of 2021, affordable cards that offer good travel insurance, several travel benefits, and generous reward points are American Express Gold ($250 annual fee), Chase Sapphire Preferred ($95 fee), Citi Premier ($95 fee), and Capital One Quicksilver Cash Rewards (no fee).

Hotels, Condos, Apartments, and Other Lodgings

Your accommodations—where you sleep, shower, and navigate with your wheelchair, cane, or crutches—are a huge part of your enjoyment of the trip. If it's a domestic trip and you're choosing the hotel yourself, look for national-brand hotels that were built since the passage of the Americans with Disabilities Act in 1990; these should be fully accessible.

The three most important features of the room are 1) the size and layout of the bathroom, especially if you need a roll-in shower; 2) location on the lobby floor, so you don't have to take an elevator to your room and you have an easy exit in case of emergency; 3) a bed with a height that makes transfers safe and that has a mattress with the correct firmness to avoid high-pressure areas on your bony prominences. It's best if the room is large enough to allow easy movement around the bed and other furniture.

Several hotel chains, such as Hilton and Marriott, have good room layouts across all price categories. For a more expensive option, Ritz-Carlton has an excellent accessible room design. Whenever possible, request a photo of the room (with dimensions) before you book. Because accessible rooms are in short supply, you should make your hotel reservation first before booking your transportation.

If you'd prefer to stay in a home rather than a hotel, there are several websites that list accessible properties for rent. The best-known are Airbnb and VRBO, which, combined, list more than two million properties, many of which are wheelchair accessible. In 2020, I searched VRBO for wheelchair-accessible two-bedroom condos and apartments that could sleep at least four people in Panama City Beach, Florida, for one week, and sixty-three listings matched my search! Many had prices of $150 to $200 per night. Even if the listing has great reviews, it's absolutely necessary to contact the owner, because the reality is that very few listings will accommodate someone with a severe disability like mine.

Domestic Air Travel

Airline reservations: Booking a flight is simple, especially with sites like Expedia or Travelocity, where you can check out the best fares and connections. Go for the first flight of the day, if possible, since it's most likely to be on time. Whenever possible, choose a nonstop flight or direct (one stop, no plane change) so you don't have to change planes. If your trip has a connecting flight, make sure the layover is at least ninety minutes. This will allow you the time to move to your next departure gate and use the restroom, if necessary.

Once you've determined an itinerary, make your flight reservations. When you receive your confirmation number, call the airline and ask to be connected with the disability or accessibility office. Some airline websites have the ability to indicate that you have a disability and require help, but often, you'll end up in the bulkhead seating in the front row. This is the worst place for me to sit, because it has no storage at your feet and no room to stretch your legs. Therefore, you should always speak to someone in reservations. They will give you preferential seating and make sure that the ground staff know that you'll be in a wheelchair and will need help boarding.

Ground transportation reservations: If you're not part of a tour, you will need to arrange for transportation from the airport to your accommodations. There are three options:

1. Rent a car or van (be sure to specify what kind of controls you need based on your abilities, and, if possible, choose the same model as the one you use at home).
2. Use the hotel shuttle or an airport shuttle that will take you to the hotel.
3. Use accessible public transportation available at the airport.

Checking in and getting to the airport: Check in online twenty-four hours before departure. For peace of mind, I like to have both a printed copy of my boarding pass and a digital copy on my phone. Even if you've purchased a ticket that doesn't include checked baggage, you'll likely not be charged to check bags that contain medical supplies and equipment. However, it is essential that you bring your medications for the entire trip with you on the plane.

Give yourself plenty of time to get to the airport, and if there's baggage service outside the terminal, use it; you'll save the trouble of carrying your baggage or finding a porter. If you have time, go to the check-in counter. The agents can help you navigate the airport, go through security, and get to your departure gate. Let them know you will need an aisle chair (the chair used to take you from the jetway into the plane; the aisle space between seats is too small for a wheelchair) to get to your seat if necessary. While you are at the counter, get new boarding passes, and get a gate check tag for your wheelchair. If the plane is large enough, and your wheelchair folds up small enough, you will be allowed to take it on the plane with you. Do *not* let the check-in counter staff take your wheelchair. If there's a problem with the plane and you need an electric chair, you could be stuck in an airport wheelchair for hours, with no seat cushion and no way to move by yourself. Even more important, you may not be able to switch flights because of the time required to move your wheelchair from one plane to the next.

Electric wheelchairs *must* be stowed in cargo, and the check-in staff will ask you what kind of battery you have. I find it useful to have a printout from the owner's manual about the battery and how to shut it off. It is important that the battery be a dry cell or gel battery, not a lead acid battery. If you have a lead acid battery, you will be in for a difficult time. The battery must be removed from your chair, placed in a secure box, and transported separately, because of the risk of the acid spilling in the cargo hold.

Going through security: The airlines are responsible for helping you get to security. Tell the ticket agent as soon as you check in that you will need assistance. There are usually two lanes at the security gate. You can use the wheelchair-accessible entrance or the TSA lane, which is usually better. It's worth spending the money ($75 in 2021) necessary to obtain a TSA Known Traveler Number (KTN). With a KTN, TSA will usually test only for explosive compounds by swabbing your chair with a small wipe. Without a KTN, TSA must perform a manual screening. In most airports, this means a complete pat-down from shoulders to feet, as well as an inspection of your pants, your chair cushion, and anything else they think is necessary. This can take up to ten minutes and is frequently intrusive and unpleasant.

Getting to the gate: Once you arrive at the departure gate, introduce yourself to the airline personnel. If you weren't able to book adjoining seats for you and your traveling companions, the gate agent may be able to change your seat assignments. Many times, they will automatically want to put you in the bulkhead, which is the first row in any class of service. But the bulkhead has no place to store items under the seat in front of you and usually doesn't have an armrest that can be lifted out of the way to make a transfer easier. Some travelers prefer the bulkhead section, though, because it means less time in the aisle chair and allows for the quickest exit.

Boarding the airplane: This should be relatively easy. Park your wheelchair at the end of the jetway, then transfer to an aisle chair. An aisle chair is a very narrow chair that can be pushed down the center aisle. Most people will be lifted from the chair into a seat. However, because the armrests raise up, you can do a sit-pivot transfer if the height of the chair and seat are similar.

It's important to bring a bag to carry wheelchair parts that might be lost or damaged from travel and handling. I usually remove my head rest, thigh guards, and joystick. I strap my seat cushion with the safety belt and leave it attached to the chair because it's too heavy to carry on the plane. If the weather report predicts rain or snow, I cover the cushion with a plastic sheet to keep it dry, since it may be transported outside to your next destination.

Enjoying the flight: Once you're onboard, enjoy the flight. Since you'll be among the first passengers on the plane, use the extra time to introduce yourself to the flight attendants. Make sure that you shift your weight every hour by leaning forward for five to ten minutes, or, if you are strong enough, pushing up as you do in your chair. If you need to go to the bathroom, call for assistance to get there. If you have a urine bag, bring along a bottle with a screw cap so that you can empty it at your seat.

Getting off the plane, retrieving your baggage, and assessing any damage: You will be among the last people off the plane, and will repeat in reverse the steps you used to get on. The crew can't leave the plane with you on it, so they will get you to your next flight or to baggage claim. If you have a tight connection, ask the flight attendant to contact the gate agent for your connecting flight. Once you've arrived at your destination, the baggage handlers will bring your wheelchair to you on the jetway so you can transfer there and move yourself to baggage claim. *Check to make sure there's no damage to your wheelchair.* The most common serious damage is to the clutch, which is disengaged to push the wheelchair manually. Frequently, the baggage handlers pull it out too far and damage the mechanism so it can no longer be pushed and, when you stop, it won't engage the brake to stop you. The plastic parts of the chair are often damaged when someone grabs them to lift the chair. Check your baggage while you are still at the airport, especially if you have a shower chair, because it's heavy and may be frequently dropped. If you find any damage, report it immediately in the baggage claim area. Take photos of the damage and make sure you have contact information for the airline's repair company.

Finding your van, car, or driver and getting to the hotel: To get to your accommodations, you have several options. The least expensive is to use public transportation such as the subway or local bus. In large cities, you can frequently arrange for a handicap-accessible taxi. Or you can rent a car or van and meet the driver outside the terminal. Your vacation has begun!

Hotels and Other Accommodations

Checking in at your hotel: When you check in at the hotel, you may experience a moment of panic if you are told that there are no accessible rooms available. This happens to me almost 50 percent of the time. This is *not* acceptable. In the US, hotels are required by the ADA to have accessible rooms, and your confirmation should show that you reserved one. Hold your ground and speak to the manager. An accessible room will magically appear!

Checking out your room: When you get to your room, check that it has all the essentials. Does it have a bathroom with a roll-in shower, enough space to turn around, a shower wand, and correct toilet height (14–18 inches/35–45 cm), as well as an acceptable bed (height and firmness) and enough room to maneuver?

Check out the key features of the hotel: Before you unpack, make sure you know the location of the fire exits, ice machine, fitness room, pool, and restaurants. Then, freshen up and introduce yourself to the concierge and the porter. The concierge can be very helpful in recommending nearby restaurants that you can roll to, accessible tourist sites, and good tours. The porter will be essential if you have rented a car or need a handicap taxi.

Enjoying Your Vacation

Meeting with your tour group: Usually, fellow members of a tour group will be staying in the same hotel, especially if the tour is designed for people with disabilities. When you check in, there should be information on where to meet for dinner or the next day's excursion. If you experience any problems, contact your tour guide or the company sponsoring the tour.

Getting around efficiently and safely: If you're not part of a tour group, the three options for transportation from the airport are the same for sightseeing at your destination. If the city has designated accessible taxis and subways, the concierge can help you with a reservation or advice on the best way to use the subway.

Keeping your routine intact: Traveling is difficult on your body's biorhythms, because the dehydration you experience in an airplane, as well as the limitations on movement, can lead to constipation and/or fatigue from lack of sleep, especially if there's a significant time-zone change. As soon as you're settled at your accommodations, devise a plan to integrate the exercise, rest, diet, and hygiene routine you follow at home.

International Air Travel

International air travel typically involves more airline rules, especially regarding carry-on luggage; keeping your wheelchair safe, because wheelchairs (especially power ones) are much less common outside the US; and passing through passport control and customs, which can be difficult with a power chair. There may be problems communicating in a different language, so it's essential that you have a printout of your detailed itinerary for taxi, shuttle, and hotel personnel to read. I frequently print the instructions on operating my wheelchair in the language of my destination country (thank goodness for Google Translate!).

Train Travel

Domestic train travel: Trains are an excellent form of travel for short trips in a wheelchair. Trains are comfortable when you're awake, but sleeping conditions on trains can be difficult, which is why I don't recommend trips of more than twenty-four hours. In a sleeping car, there are usually upper and lower berths, which are difficult to transfer into and have mattresses that can cause unwanted pressure. If your destination is more than twenty-four hours away by train, consider other forms of transportation instead.

International train travel: Because many trains in Europe and Asia are high-speed, it's rare that a trip will take more than ten or twelve hours. These trains have advantages over planes in that they usually bring you to the center of the city, which is more convenient. They are frequently less expensive than flying and avoid many of the security issues found in airports. If possible, upgrade from economy to first class, because you'll have more room and better service for food and drink.

Bus Tours

Local sightseeing tours: Almost all major cities have accessible bus tours; the concierge at your hotel can provide you with information, but I also suggest researching in advance. Big Bus Tours and City Sightseeing, for example, have tours in more than fifty cities. Many cities have made public buses wheelchair-accessible. In others, all buses are equipped with a ramp or a lift, and some cities have a separate fleet of wheelchair-accessible buses that can be accessed by calling the public transit office. The major advantage of using public transportation is that the cost is by far the lowest of any transportation mode; usually it's the same for disabled and nondisabled passengers. If you plan to stay in one city for several days, you can usually purchase a multi-day pass that is good for three to seven days, allowing you to make several sightseeing trips at a low cost.

Multi-city tours: There are many companies that offer accessible tours similar to the ones they offer for nondisabled travelers. Bus tours are frequently much less expensive than other disability tours because they share the same tour guides and facilities. They also tend to use less-expensive hotels and restaurants. For sightseeing in a city, they are particularly cost-effective, since you won't need to take taxis from place to place.

Domestic Car Travel

The pack-up-the-car-and-family-and-head-west trip has been a long-standing tradition in the US, and it remains one of the least expensive ways to travel. Plus, it gives you great flexibility to spend more or less time in any place along the way. You may consider visiting and/or staying at any of the national parks.

The biggest problem with road trips is that, at 65 mph (105 km/h), it takes a long time to get to your destination, which can be difficult for people with disabilities. I limit my car travel to about six hours at a time, because longer trips cause me too much pain and stiffness. Also, you might have to do most of the trip planning and hotel booking yourself, unless you are an AAA member or you have a travel agent.

International Car Travel

Traveling by car in other countries is usually OK, but it's not great. The major problem is a lack of accessible cars and vans. If you're able to find one, the cost is usually much higher than it is at home. Also, navigating is difficult, even with GPS. Parking can be difficult, too, because vans are much larger than most cars and there are very few accessible parking spaces.

Cruises

Cruises are a preferred mode of vacation travel for many people with disabilities. The greatest benefit is that you don't have to pack up and change hotels during your vacation. You stay put and let the ship travel from place to place. Cruises also offer a wide selection of travel possibilities in terms of cost, duration, places to visit, amenities, food, entertainment, and flexibility. Recently, more cruise lines have been offering accessible rooms, which are larger than standard rooms, and land excursions designed for people with significant disabilities. My wife and I enjoy cruises because they are easy to schedule, you can easily make new friends, the food and entertainment are usually excellent, and the newer ships are easy to navigate in a wheelchair. Most times, the only drawback is the size of the room, which is often smaller than an accessible hotel room. But if you're willing to forgo an upper-deck cabin or to accept one with no view, you can purchase a cruise at a very competitive price compared to other types of travel.

Emergencies

Medical emergencies are one of the most feared problems you may encounter while traveling. Travel can make you susceptible to illness because of stress, changes in time zone, altered diet, dehydration, and sleep deprivation. If you're traveling in a developed country, there should be good emergency care nearby, and most medical and minor surgical problems can be handled well at any local hospital.

More complex surgery for critical care emergency problems should be taken care of at hospitals with specialized services. This is especially true if you have a stroke, because only comprehensive stroke centers can mobilize the medical team, sophisticated imaging, and therapeutic techniques needed to limit stroke damage. If you're in a major city, this type of care will be readily available; if you're in a rural area, the best course of action is to be transported by air (usually by helicopter) to the nearest critical care hospital. The situation is similar for SCI and TBI. There are hospitals with special teams and technology designated as level one trauma centers, where you should be transported as quickly as possible.

If you're traveling internationally, the situation can be much more complicated. If you're in a developing country, the likely course of action is for you to be taken to the nearest hospital for assessment. If you are critically ill, you should be airlifted to the nearest critical care hospital. A list of medical air ambulances is included in the Resources section, but usually your insurer will dictate which vendor to use. The cost of an air ambulance ($30,000 to $50,000, as of 2021) is usually covered in part by your medical insurance. You will also likely have the additional expense of being taken care of in a hospital by doctors who are "out of network," which can leave you with a bill in the tens of thousands of dollars. This is the moment you'll be glad that you purchased travel insurance to help cover the cost.

Keep Exploring

If traveling was important to you before your injury, I encourage you to find ways to continue that activity as your rehabilitation allows. Start with destinations close to home and get comfortable with the new normal of travel protocols for you before venturing farther out.

Everything You Need to Know

Travel after ANI is more difficult and requires more planning and more attention to detail. Unless you must travel internationally to see family, it's best to make your first few vacations domestic ones. That way, you don't have to deal with a language barrier, different laws, and an unknown health care system, should the need arise. You'll also be spending less time in an airplane. Most important, you'll be developing tactics that make for a smooth experience on future trips; through trial and error, you'll learn what works best for you.

No matter your destination, be sure to carry with you print and digital copies of every detail regarding your reservations, including the carrier, your accommodations, transportation at your destination, and tour details. Travel will get easier for you with each trip you make. And although getting to your destination will be less carefree than it used to be, I guarantee it's worth the effort.

18

You Are *Not* Invisible

How to Thrive in Your Community

ALTHOUGH IT SEEMED FARFETCHED while I was lying in bed on a ventilator, almost completely paralyzed, I still had a lot to offer. You do too. During rehabilitation, make sure this goal is on your short list: returning as an active participant in community life. This vision of yourself will enhance your recovery and help you strengthen vital connections beyond your immediate family.

There are four things to consider as you integrate back into your community: friends, employment and finances, advocacy, and helping others.

1. **Friends are essential to a satisfying life, and no doubt you have enjoyed the enrichment of long-lasting friendships over the years.** As odd as it may seem, after your injury, you may wonder where your friends have gone. Just when you need them the most, they seem to have disappeared. What's up?

   The fact is, if you are unable to speak due to your injury, have difficulty speaking clearly enough to be understood, or have trouble understanding what others are saying to you, your friends may be so uncomfortable at seeing your disability—and not knowing how to "be" with this new version of you—that they will shy away from visiting. Or, if your injury has left you in a wheelchair, fully or partially paralyzed, friends may be at a loss as to how to interact with you, especially if your friendship revolved around activities such as hiking, hunting, skiing, and so on.

If this is the case, you'll have to take the lead. Reach out to friends and invite them to visit you at your home. Or make plans to meet at a coffee shop you both like. If the weather is nice, maybe you'll want to meet at a local park. Find a way to let your friends know that even with your new disability, you are still you—the person who loves supporting your favorite football team, or watching romantic comedies, or hanging out at the lake. Let your friends know that you understand it might feel awkward right now, but that will change with time. You may have to find new activities to enjoy together, so be open to making suggestions. Explain that you are in rehab and hope that you will continue to make progress toward a way of life that resembles the one you were leading before your injury. Put your friends at ease; sometimes asking questions like *What do you want to know about my life in a wheelchair?* is the icebreaker your friend needs. Mailing a handwritten letter may be a good first step toward reconnecting. You'll know the best approach. And, as you reach out to friends, enlist the help of your family when needed.

Joining a support group can be helpful too. You can learn how others in the group are maintaining old friendships. They, too, will have experienced that "where did everybody go?" moment. Finding out what works for others will give you some ideas you may not have considered for trying to reconnect with your friends.

There will be some friendships that just don't survive. And, while that's sad, I have some good news for you. Your injury will allow you to meet new friends (more about that later in this chapter), folks you never would have met otherwise and who will enrich your life tremendously.

After the devastation of your injury, the effort to maintain friendships and forge new ones may be a difficult task at first, but if you keep trying, you will see results. Sustaining friendships and other meaningful connections is as essential to your recovery as anything modern medicine can do for you. Don't underestimate the power of your support system. That team includes your work colleagues as well.

2. **Your work is an important place to find connection with others, even though you may not socialize with them outside the workplace.** Your job may be how you earn a living, but it's also directly tied to your self-esteem and your community. It adds structure and purpose to your day, and can benefit your mental health. Work provides

you with a built-in network of friends and colleagues, some of whom may be part of your social life. And, of course, returning to work is also fundamental to your financial health. Having a job means not only that you can support yourself and your family but that it's likely you have employer-provided health insurance, which is critical for obtaining the ongoing health care and rehabilitation services you need.

Returning to work is a big step toward getting your life back after your injury. Depending on the physical demands of your job, you may be able to return; if not, you'll need to learn new skills for a new career. During discharge planning, ask to meet with local vocational rehabilitation services to discuss your job opportunities. Establish a strong working relationship with your vocational rehabilitation counselor so that they understand your employment interests and can match you with appropriate opportunities. If discharge planning is too early for this kind of referral, you can ask your social worker or therapy team for a referral to a career counselor when you are further along in your rehabilitation. After a traumatic injury, some health insurance plans will cover this kind of counseling; disability insurance plans almost always do. These professionals can help you by identifying opportunities that you might not have thought of and showing you how to get the necessary training.

Find programs that train people with disabilities to transition to new careers. Your local community center is one place to start, as are your local colleges, universities, and vocational schools. If you don't have a college degree (associate or bachelor's), you may consider acquiring (or finishing) one; statistics show that college graduates have far greater employment opportunities and that your earning potential will double or triple. You may choose to attend a community college class (frequently available online) before enrolling in a fulltime degree program. The experience will inform you of your ability to learn (which may have changed after your injury), and your physical endurance (my arms and hands are too weak to take notes, for example, so I either use a scribe or record the lecture).

If training or more education is what you need to enter a new field, find out as soon as possible if your disability insurance policy will be sufficient to pay for it, or if your employer has funds for that kind of expense. At the same time, begin the process of applying for SSDI

(Social Security Disability Income) and SSI (Supplemental Security Income); both of these have programs that will support you while you train for a new job. The Social Security Administration's Plan to Achieve Self-Support (PASS) program is designed to help you pay for items necessary to search for work, such as wheelchairs and computers. Note: You must apply for, or already receive, Supplemental Security Income (SSI) benefits to qualify for the PASS program. You may also be able to continue receiving SSDI while you are transitioning to employment using Social Security's Ticket to Work program.

If you're having trouble paying bills, medical or otherwise, before you return to work, there are a number of additional programs and organizations that can help. The Patient Advocate Foundation is a national organization that can help you 1) negotiate bills with hospitals, doctors, and insurance companies; 2) access rehabilitation organizations; and 3) handle any issues with a previous or new employer. It's a well-run and highly charitable organization that assists many people with disabilities and chronic illnesses. You may also want to investigate local foundations and community health programs (you'll find more information in the Resources section on page 283).

If you won't be able to return to your old job, and it included a health insurance plan that paid for prescription drugs, you may still be able to access those prescriptions through prescription assistance programs, which most pharmaceutical companies will offer. These programs provide free or low-cost drugs to uninsured people who are unable to afford their medications. The Partnership for Prescription Assistance is another resource; a clearinghouse for more than 475 public and private assistance programs, it includes nearly 200 pharmaceutical options. RxAssist, NeedyMeds, and many others (see Resources, page 284) offer steep discounts on drugs and prescription drug discount cards.

If your injury makes it impossible for you to return to work or to train for a new occupation, Social Security has funds for those who are permanently disabled. Your social worker will help you with the necessary applications. But even if you're unable to work again after your injury, you can still be a valued member of your community. Advocacy and volunteer opportunities are rewarding ways for you to connect with others beyond your family and friends.

3. **Advocacy: Support the local disability community in whatever ways you can.** Grassroots advocacy is an important part of how citizens affect changes to our society. It's an effective way to be involved in the development of the laws and policies that affect our lives—to make our voices heard. It was through the advocacy of folks like you and me that the ADA became law, greatly improving quality of life for those with disabilities. The ADA made us *visible*. Laws that made it possible for us to enjoy public places with nondisabled people helped us, our families, and our communities in too many ways to count.

There are many ways to be an advocate. If you've joined a support group, there may be members who are also part of a local chapter of a larger advocacy organization or who can point you in the right direction. Disability advocacy groups work to improve rights and access for people with disabilities, but they may focus on more specific causes; these may be access to education, or to equipment, or to work, or to another area where there's a need.

There are many advocacy groups to choose from; some of the larger ones with a national presence include ADA Watch, a project of the National Coalition for Disability Rights; Americans Disabled for Attendant Programs Today (ADAPT), a national grassroots community that works to assure the civil and human rights of people with disabilities; the American Association of People with Disabilities (AAPD), a national voice for change in implementing the goals of the ADA; and the Patient Advocate Foundation (PAF), which is particularly useful for negotiating business issues related to access to care, medical debt, and job retention. You'll find a list in the Resources section on page 284.

As part of your advocacy, be sure you are registered to vote in your state. Ask for an absentee ballot, because sometimes your voting site isn't accessible or the weather isn't conducive to traveling to the polls.

Attend an Advocacy Day event. These are organized by state and bring together groups of people with specific ANIs to raise awareness of their issues and advocate for public policy initiatives. These events are a great opportunity to make your voice heard in your state legislature and provide a time to meet your local representatives in person.

Your elected officials, and those legislators in position to change policy, need to hear directly from you, so it's important that you learn about the legislative process. The local and national advocacy groups that you belong to will establish a list of priority policies that they believe will have the greatest impact on the quality of life of their members. Your advocacy group can assist you in finding your representatives in the House of Representatives and Senate. If you have the opportunity during Advocacy Day, or if and when you happen to be in Washington, DC, arrange a visit to your representative's office to meet in person. There's nothing quite like face-to-face interaction to convey the importance of an issue.

My Advocacy Efforts

I've focused my advocacy efforts at the state level. Specifically, there are two programs in New York State that support fundamental and translational research relevant to ANI. The first is the New York State Stem Cell Funding Board (NYSTEM) that provides up to $60 million dollars yearly to support research on stem cells in New York. I was fortunate to be chosen by a local politician to be on the NYSTEM Committee, which enables me to advocate for stem cell research at all levels of government. The second is the Spinal Cord Injury Research Board, which provides $8.5 million for SCI research. I've advocated with several local state representatives to continue this funding that has made New York one of the best states in which to perform SCI research.

4. **Helping others: By helping others, you can find a positive way to integrate back into the community.** You may be thinking: *Helping others? I'm in need of help myself!* Yes, your life has new difficulties, but there are still opportunities to help others in need. As you do, you will continue to nurture your resilience.

Volunteer to be a mentor at a local school or as one of the children's story-hour readers at your local library. Your local community center or senior center is usually looking for people who can volunteer to teach a class on a one-time basis or once a week for six weeks, for example; perhaps you can give a presentation on gardening in small spaces, or savvy investing strategies, or writing poetry, or taking nature photos—wherever your interests lie. Food pantries are always in need of volunteers, and so are hospitals. Perhaps you'd like to spend three hours a week at the patient information desk, or in the hospital gift shop, or the coffee shop. The opportunities are as limitless as your interests and imagination.

Perhaps you would like to participate in a local organization that does charitable work. Find a chapter of the General Federation of Women's Clubs, Lions Club International, Rotary International, or another well-established group. Once you've attended a few meetings, you'll figure out what kind of role you want to play in their efforts to support members of the community.

In my city, the Rochester Spinal Association (RSA) has a monthly support group that includes a one-hour social event, followed by a one-hour presentation on a topic of broad interest. The RSA provides members with an opportunity to express their feelings, learn helpful information, improve social skills, and realize they are not alone. It's also a good place to network—about jobs, doctors, new adaptive sports programs, grants for equipment and therapy, and new therapists, including those for acupuncture, massage, yoga, and tai chi. Most important, through its fundraising efforts, the RSA provides grants to help ANI survivors purchase assistive equipment, get health care if they lack insurance, and improve their quality of life by providing access to fitness, nutrition, and smoking cessation programs.

You can help with fundraising—volunteers are always needed. And being part of an effort to raise money to help people with disabilities enjoy a better life is rewarding. While the amount of money your local organizations distribute may be small, the impact it has on the people who receive the funds is enormous. Through your participation, you're not only helping people but also helping increase general awareness of the challenges that people with ANI face. And, you'll be making many new friends.

Whenever I'm out at a social event—at dinner, a play, a music performance—people tell me that I'm an "inspiration." I've learned that my positive outlook, willingness to be seen in public, and improvement in function over the years makes them believe they can achieve the same recovery from their own severe injury or illness. At first, I was embarrassed by this attention, but I've learned to embrace it and pay it forward. I believe that my presence sends a message: If you hire someone with a disability, work with someone with a disability, or are able to help someone with a disability, you will understand how talented and capable they are. Or, if you are that person with a disability, I'm hopeful that my example will give you a more positive outlook on your own ability to be a valued member of your community. So, go ahead: Be an inspiration.

You are just as worthy after your injury as you were before it. When you establish yourself as an active member of your community, you foster connections that show you just how significant your role is—as a friend, a colleague, a mentor, an advocate, or a volunteer.

———

Everything You Need to Know

After ANI, you may feel like retreating to a hermit-like existence. But, trust me, you'll feel so much better if you resist those thoughts and put yourself out there. Find a way to reconnect with friends and to get back to work or transition to a new type of employment. Become an advocate for others with a disability and find a way to help those in need in your community.

It's important for you as well as for members of your community that you remain an active participant in social and civic affairs. Living with a disability does not mean you no longer have meaningful contributions to make—you can develop a role as an advocate, as a mentor, and as a person who cares about quality of life in the community at large. These activities will add meaning to your daily life.

Turn to friends and family members to help you reenter community life, and be emboldened to try membership in organizations you previously thought were too pedestrian for you (or perhaps too elite). Use your new status to become more outgoing. You'll enjoy how this shift in approaching strangers in your community transforms your life.

Our quality of life is enhanced by our connections with others. Your willingness and determination to become and remain a visible person in your community will bring joy not only to your own life but also to your family and to a long list of strangers who will become trusted friends.

Future Therapies

Science and Technology Bring the Future
to the Now

Y RECOVERY FROM A severe SCI has been remarkable—I've regained far more function than I initially thought possible, and my recovery is ongoing; it continues to this day.

Of course, there are other stories out there like mine that defy what we *think* we know to be the limits of possibility. What I believe now, based on my experience and research, is that we've barely scratched the surface of what there is to learn about the potential for recovery from an acute neurological injury. As I look at the horizon in this field of medicine, I'm convinced we will see remarkable advances over the next ten years.

These promising therapies share a common theme: They take advantage of the intrinsic capacity of neurons that were spared from injury and the connections they make (called "circuits," because they work like the components of modern electronics) to produce movement and sensation. This phenomenon is the foundation of neuroplasticity, which can be enhanced by "high-intensity therapy" to help these circuits reorganize and stimulate recovery.

There are five areas of research and development where I believe the most important advances will occur:

1. **Devices:** Robots, exoskeletons, nerve stimulators (epidural electrical stimulation [EES] and transcutaneous electrical stimulation [TCS] of the spinal cord), brain-computer interfaces (BCI), scaffolds for nerve regeneration, and adaptive and recreational devices.

2. **Neuroplasticity enhanced by drugs and devices:** Devices and drugs to promote neuroplasticity by improving learning, sensory

and motor integration, and substitution of one sensory modality for another (like substituting touch—Braille—for vision to read).

3. **Regenerative medicine:** Stem cell mobilization, differentiation, and transplantation; induced pluripotent stem cells (iPSC); and drugs and scaffolds to promote nerve regeneration.

4. **Integrative medicine:** Understanding the mechanisms by which complementary therapies such as acupuncture, probiotics, and traditional Chinese medicine work to provide a rich source of new treatments and improved use of these ancient therapies.

5. **Clinical trials:** An explosion of clinical trials will offer patients the opportunity to test new therapies in a highly regulated environment that involves little or no risk. If the treatment is beneficial, the volunteer might recover important functions such as improved strength and sensation.

Devices

When we look to the future in neurorestoration, my money is on devices. I'm confident that, five years from now, I'll have dramatically increased my independence because of new devices that are being developed, refined, and tested right now.

Motor devices: Moving an arm or leg requires your brain to send electrical signals to your limb's muscles, causing them to contract. Neuroscientists call these "move signals." The part of the brain known as the primary motor cortex helps to calculate the move signals for the limb (Figure 1, see page 10). At the same time, the brain needs to receive signals from the arm or leg telling you where the limb is located relative to the rest of your body and to other objects nearby, as observed by your eyes. This information is then integrated using the sensorimotor cortex and other regions of the brain that monitor balance and touch through a process called sensorimotor integration.

A device that can perform these tasks needs to be highly sophisticated. One way to simplify the process is to take advantage of the nerves that are alive in the arm and leg, as well as in the brain. In theory, these nerves can be reactivated or rerouted to fill the need. There are already several devices capable of performing these tasks and clear paths toward developing even better technologies.

Walking rehabilitation and epidural electric stimulation (EES): One of the most significant disabilities experienced by people with ANI is the inability to walk. If you have a complete SCI above S1, you will have difficulty walking; if you have a TBI or stroke that causes significant damage to the motor or sensory regions of the cortex that innervate the lower limbs, walking will be impaired in proportion to the extent of your injury.

These observations support the theory that these injuries would have no recovery of function, since there's no connection from the brain to the muscles and nerves below. But in 2011, this belief was shown to be incorrect when a twenty-three-year-old man with complete paraplegia (an SCI from C7 to T1) regained the ability to stand and perform stepping movements voluntarily.[1]

He performed 170 locomotor training sessions over twenty-six months, and then a sixteen-electrode array was placed on the dura (outer covering of the spinal cord that covered the L1 to S1 cord segments) to enable epidural electrical stimulation (EES) of the nerves in that region (Figure 38A, similar to Figure 13; see page 82). The investigators adjusted the stimulation protocol to optimize standing and stepping (Figure 38B). At optimal settings, he was able to stand with minimal assistance and could make stepping-like movements when the settings were optimized for

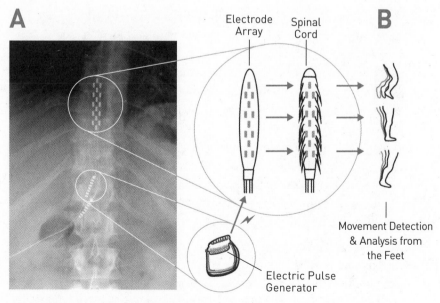

Figure 38. EES restoration of walking in SCI

movement. Even more exciting: After seven months, he regained some voluntary control of his legs, although it required EES.

This success with intense rehabilitation and EES therapy shows that the spinal cord is smart; it can use sensory information to produce a coordinated movement without input from the brain. This proves that the spinal cord contains circuits that are not normally used, called central pattern generators (CPGs). CPGs can produce simple movements such as stepping and enable postures like standing.

There have been three major recent advances in the field since 2011:

1. The stimulation protocols have been optimized to allow more sensory signals to activate the spinal cord.[2] The goal is to reproduce the natural activation of the spinal cord sensory and motor nerves and, in people with incomplete SCI, to send information to the brain.[3]

2. Patients with SCI were treated within *one week of their injury* using EES that was delivered to specific nerve bundles in the lumbosacral spinal cord, at a frequency that matched the intended movement. Within one week, this protocol reestablished control of paralyzed muscles during overground walking that improved during rehabilitation. Most impressive, after a few months, the patients regained voluntary control over their paralyzed muscles *without stimulation.*[4]

3. Transcutaneous spinal cord stimulation was shown to improve the speed and quality of walking for people with chronic (>1 year) incomplete SCI.[5] This noninvasive therapy in patients with chronic SCI offers potential benefits to thousands of people with SCI. It also suggests that similar approaches could be used to restore upper-limb paralysis and could be used in people with stroke as well.

During these studies, some people also showed improvement in blood pressure, as well as bowel, bladder, and sexual function. Sometimes these improvements were permanent, even after the stimulators were turned off.[6] These successes point to fantastic possibilities to improve the autonomic and sympathetic nervous systems in all ANIs as we look to the future.

Exoskeletons: The concept for exoskeletons has been around since 1917. Designing and building practical exoskeletons, however, has proved difficult. The first FDA-approved exoskeleton was the ReWalk exoskeleton for everyday use (Figure 29A). The same company, ReWalk Robotics,

Optimization of EES to Obtain Normal Sensorimotor Integration for Walking

To be successful, EES must occur in the correct physical location in the spinal cord and at the correct time during the three phases of a single step (Figure 38B). The figure shows a sixteen-electrode array attached to an electrical pulse generator to stimulate the nerves. Several electrodes are activated to stimulate specific groups of nerves beginning with the swing phase (phase 1), followed by a different set of electrodes activated during weight acceptance (phase 2), and finally, another set activated during propulsion forward (phase 3).[7] Scientifically, the process is an algorithm for EES stimulation that matches the location and timing of natural motor neuron activation. (An algorithm is a series of mathematical formulas that describe the information necessary to perform a specific movement, such as bending your knee.) Another algorithm that measures real-time foot movements can adjust the location and timing of the stimulation protocols to your current environment.

has also developed an exoskeleton called ReStore for stroke patients, which assists a single leg and synchronizes the gait with the other leg (Figure 29B). Bodyweight-assisted exoskeletons and the ReWalk are beneficial for regaining normal gait, balance, and the strength necessary for safe and efficient walking. Currently, these devices are expensive and can be cumbersome. But the future holds more sophisticated designs, lightweight materials, and better functional capabilities.

Neuroprosthetics: Almost everyone with ANI could benefit from specialized neuroprosthetics that incorporate lightweight exoskeleton technology. For example, I would like to kayak again, but I'm unable to do so because of my limited upper-extremity strength. A lightweight neuroprosthesis designed just for my arms that is waterproof, easy to put on, and adjustable to facilitate the motions of paddling would be extremely useful. This would be similar to a balanced forearm orthosis (Figure 34), except that it can strengthen your weak arm and hold on to tools and recreational objects. Developing platforms that contain interchangeable components for specific muscles and joints, which can be easily individualized with 3D printing, would be helpful for anyone with an ANI. Continuous rehab is essential to maximize your recovery. I believe that use of these devices will be a cost-effective means to promote neuroplasticity and functional recovery.

Sensory Devices

We rely on constant input from different types of sensory cells (mechanoreceptors, photoreceptors, chemoreceptors, thermoreceptors) in specialized organs to obtain real-time information about our environment. Signals from sensory organs travel to the spinal cord and then to the sensory areas in the brain, where they are processed and interpreted (except for cranial, olfactory, optic, and trigeminal nerves that are more accurately considered part of the central nervous system). Multiple sensations are frequently integrated to create a perceptual experience. For example, I enjoy good wine. The perceptual experience is a combination of the color of the wine, the smell of the bouquet, the multiple tastes I perceive when I swirl it in my mouth, and the flavor that it generates when combined with food. Many of the things we enjoy most stimulate multiple sensory organs and create unique experiences.

Hearing and speech are the top two disabilities after ANI, because they prevent communication and social interactions, the psychological mainstays of our existence.

Hearing: For people with ANI, especially stroke and TBI, loss of hearing may be so profound that even hearing aids aren't satisfactory. One option is to use a cochlear implant, which bypasses the lower parts of the brain and acts as a neuroprosthesis to restore hearing.[8] It replaces the normal hearing process with electric signals that directly stimulate the auditory nerve. If you receive a cochlear implant and intense auditory training, you should be able to interpret these auditory signals as sound and speech.[9] Future devices to enable hearing will likely be less invasive and deliver even better hearing.

Vision: Loss of vision is primarily a problem for people whose stroke or TBI has damaged the part of the brain that contains the visual cortex (Figure 1, occipital lobe). When this occurs on one side of your brain, you lose vision in the opposite field of view proportionate to the size of the stroke. This blind spot creates a large area that cannot be seen without turning your head, which leads to an increased propensity for falls and accidents when driving. But there's strong evidence that, after sufficient time and practice, the injured brain can learn to see again. People with blindsight can recover their vision, and we have the ability to respond to images that we don't consciously see (see Figure 7, page 45).

With intense practice, you can learn to be aware of and process these images, using a computerized learning program that is individualized for you. Learning takes a lot of time, so to accelerate learning, there have been trials of both drugs and devices. A 2019 clinical trial showed that a noninvasive electrical current, transcranial random noise stimulation (tRNS), had remarkable effects to speed up recovery of vision.[10] Translation of this technology into clinical practice will likely take several years, but it offers more rapid and greater recovery of sight for people who have damaged their occipital lobe and visual cortex.

Position, motion, and temperature: These three senses are part of the somatosensory system, which also includes perception of touch, pressure, temperature, and vibration. The nerves that comprise the somatosensory system are frequently damaged after an ANI, either in the brain (stroke or TBI) or in the spinal cord (SCI). Several studies have shown that sensation-specific training (e.g., repetitive exposure to liquids of different temperature, movement of fingers and toes) combined with stimulation by transcranial random noise stimulation (tRNS) or transcranial magnetic stimulation (TMS) can significantly improve many kinds of sensation.[11] Examples include fine motion of your hands to enable you to button up a shirt, thread a needle, drive a car, type and use a mouse on your computer, and play video games.

Pain: Pain, or nociception, is perceived by the stimulation of sensory nerves. Devices that control pain usually involve spinal cord stimulation (SCS; Figure 13, see page 82). SCS refers here to a basic type of EES in which the 16-electrode array is placed in the thoracolumbar region to block pain from that region. Placement in the cervical region is possible but has more risks because cranial nerves exit from the cervical spinal cord. SCS relieves pain in people with ANI, as well as people with spinal stenosis and arthritis, by masking pain signals with electrical signals that block nerve impulses from nociceptive nerves. These devices are FDA-approved for treatment of chronic pain of the trunk, limbs, and low back, and for complex regional pain syndrome (CRPS). Over the last ten years, new kinds of stimulation have made SCS more effective and safer, including wireless systems, miniaturization, and better electrodes. This area of medicine will continue to improve in efficacy and safety in the future and become less invasive.

Advanced Technology Devices

Brain-computer interfaces (BCI): BCI is the most sophisticated technology to help people with paralysis. It's still in a highly experimental state and will likely not be commercially available for several years. BCI comprises: 1) electrodes implanted in the brain's motor cortex, under the skull over the dura, or on the skull itself like an EEG electrode, which detect electrical signals while you think of a desired movement; 2) a computer interface to decode the signals into machine language that enables computers to process the information; 3) transmission of the information to a neuroprosthesis such as a robotic arm or hand, or to an exoskeleton such as the balanced forearm orthosis (Figure 36) and, ultimately, to nerves and/or muscles that respond to the signal; and 4) a sensory device that provides feedback on the resulting movement.

The current state of development has resulted in devices that enable a person with paraplegia to operate a BCI-robotic arm, which controls reach and grasp movements. But these BCI devices require invasive electrodes in which the skull is opened and the electrodes are implanted into the brain tissue, so they aren't useful for the long term. In 2019, a French study reported the use of a BCI implanted between the skull and the dura (which covers the brain) for twenty-four months. A tetraplegic man used the device to control a virtual avatar, and in the laboratory he controlled a four-limbed exoskeleton to make stepping movements, although he required bodyweight support for balance.[12] This provides the strongest evidence to date that BCI technology can become safe, durable, and functional in everyday life. The development of electrodes that are less invasive, similar to those used for EEGs, will improve the transition of BCI from the laboratory to the community.

Artificial intelligence (AI): AI will become an important tool for neurorehabilitation, because the algorithms that will be developed to decode information from the sensorimotor cortex will be individualized, which should enable more accurate and efficient movement. When multiple algorithms are put together, a complete movement, such as reach and grasp, is obtained. The results from hundreds or even thousands of users will be analyzed by scientists and AI experts to identify key patterns that can be used to optimize routine movements such as opening a door or jar, reaching for and grasping a glass, or grasping and pulling a zipper. Using these standard algorithms, AI will then analyze your unique data to create an algorithm that is specific for you, based on your own muscle strength, flexibility, and range of motion.

Speech synthesis: Speech synthesis is the artificial production of human speech. Fifteen years ago, this would have been a heroic achievement, but today almost 1 billion people worldwide routinely use smart speakers such as Siri (Apple), Alexa (Amazon), and OK Google (Android) to request information and enable dictation. The future will bring us the "Internet of Things," a network of physical objects—"things"—that are embedded with sensors, software, and other technologies to connect and exchange data with control devices over the Internet. Currently the "smart home" uses devices such as smartphones and smart speakers to control lights, thermostats, and home security systems. For those of us with ANI limitations, this technology will offer almost unlimited accessibility and interaction with our environment. Perhaps the last frontier will be to combine this technology with electrical signal recordings in the brain to enable speech production and speech recognition for stroke and TBI survivors who have sufficient damage to make verbal communication impossible.

Adaptive and Recreational Devices

Sports and recreational activities: After ANI, sporting activities can be difficult, primarily because of the following limitations: 1) decreased range of motion, poor strength, and lack of sensation in the upper extremities, especially the hands; 2) poor balance due to a lack of core strength; and 3) paralysis of the lower limbs requiring the use of wheelchairs for movement. Improving upper-extremity function is the most difficult problem, because the range of motion required for normal function is so great. Currently, there are task-specific adaptive technologies that can assist with simple movements, such as rotating your hand and swinging your arm forward. However, it will require BCI technology to achieve upper-extremity strength and range of motion to participate in sports like tennis or golf. The problems with improving balance and core strength are similar. Neuroprosthetics that are universal in terms of range of motion and strength but adjustable to the demands of a specific sport are the hope of the future. I think it's also likely that improvements in exoskeleton and epidural electrical stimulation technology will have significant crossover benefits for sports and recreation.

The biggest change recently has been dramatic improvements in wheel-chair technology that enable people with ANI to move rapidly in one direction. It's still difficult to change direction, especially when going back-ward, and there's also significant overuse of the shoulder, causing damage to the rotator cuff. Because so many sports and recreational activities require movements that are multidirectional and require the use of both hands, wheelchair movement represents a great opportunity for the use of BCI technology. Specifically, the ability to think of movements that are then carried out by servomotors like those present in exoskeletons will enable an "intuitive" hands-free approach to mobility. This advance will allow you to use both hands for sports. For recreation, the ability to hike, or climb over rough terrain, using a "smart" wheelchair, will be possible using intel-ligent controls similar to self-driving cars and advances in battery power and weight that improve the distance you can travel.

Transportation: In the future, the widespread use of self-driving vehi-cles will enable almost everyone with an ANI to "drive." The only lim-itation will be getting in and out of vehicles.

Regenerative Medicine

Stem Cell Mobilization, Differentiation, and Transplants

What is a stem cell? There are several kinds of stem cells that all share two properties: self-renewal and differentiation. Self-renewal is the abil-ity of cells to grow without losing the ability to differentiate. Differen-tiation is the ability of stem cells to change into specialized cells that make up adult tissues, such as neurons, astrocytes, and microglial cells in the brain, which each perform specific functions. Stem cells can be obtained from human embryos or adult tissues by culturing the cells in special growth media. They also can be made in the laboratory by genet-ically reprogramming a differentiated, specialized cell to become similar to embryonic stem cells. For example, skin cells called fibroblasts are injected with powerful proteins known as transcription factors, which are similar to factors found during embryonic development. Stem cells made by this technique are called induced pluripotent stem cells (iPSCs). Since these cells can be obtained from the person who will be transplanted with them (autologous donation), immune compatibility is greatly increased.

What is nerve regeneration? Nerve regeneration refers to the regrowth or repair of neurons after injury. More broadly, it encompasses the regeneration of nervous tissue, which includes support cells such as glia, astrocytes, and oligodendrocytes. Stem cells provide a unique resource to regenerate nervous tissue because they are similar to the cells present in embryonic development that formed the complex nervous tissue that is the brain and spinal cord. The alternative approach of transplanting mature specialized cells and expecting them to "self-organize" into functional nervous tissue is unlikely to be successful.

Challenges in the clinical use of stem cells for tissue regeneration. The concept of using stem cells to restore dead or damaged nerve cells looks promising, based on animal studies. But six major concerns must be addressed before human tissue-specific stem cell transplants can occur:

1. **Incorporation of stem cells into tissues requires an environment that provides the stem cells with information about their correct location and interactions with other cells in the tissue.**

2. **The timing of stem cell transplants may be important.** In people with ANI, there may be a window of only one or two days immediately after the injury for a successful transplant due to inflammation and scar formation.

3. **Production of sufficient numbers of stem cells to "fill in" the space left behind may be difficult, especially for iPSCs, which can no longer grow once they differentiate.**

4. **Making transplanted stem cells differentiate into fully mature tissue.** While the cells may appear to be appropriately differentiated, they may not function properly after transplantation.

5. **There are significant concerns that the transplanted cells may not remain differentiated.** In particular, making iPSCs currently requires the use of tumor-promoting transcription factors that are transferred into cells using viruses. These viruses and factors are known to cause mutations in your DNA and increase cell growth, potentially causing cancer.

6. **Consistent stem cell production may be technically difficult, making the success rate low even prior to transplant.**

What you should know before being treated with stem cells: The stem cell field is still very new; all legitimate stem cell transplants for people with ANI are currently being given only in clinical trials. These trials, known as phase 1–2 trials, are designed to test safety and proper dose. While it's possible to obtain clinical benefit as measured by improved movement of a paralyzed limb, the trial is not designed for that purpose. Instead, the phase 3 trial is designed to test efficacy. A phase 3 trial is usually a randomized, placebo-controlled trial using the optimal dose and timing, based on results from the phase 1–2 trials. There has been one successful phase 3 trial of stem cells in seventy patients with SCI,[13] so this treatment is still many years away from clinical use. There are clinics, however, that offer (for large fees, frequently), unproven stem cell therapies. *None of these clinics are using stem cells that have proven efficacy or FDA approval.* Before you consider such a treatment, you should ask these questions: What are the anticipated benefits and how do you measure them? What's the mechanism? How are the stem cells made? What are the side effects and risks? Will you provide me with contact information to speak with people you have treated?

What are my options for participating in a stem cell trial, and will I benefit? The best way to find stem cell trials that are located near you and are actively recruiting participants is to visit clinicaltrials.gov. More than twenty-five trials have used injections of stem cells to treat ANI. The vast majority of these trials used bone marrow–derived mesenchymal stem cells (BM-MSCs) which are cells from the patient's own bone marrow. Their use in cell therapy is primarily to stimulate the intrinsic regenerative properties of injured tissues by releasing growth and differentiation factors, not by making new tissue themselves. Among the MSC trials for SCI, eight out of ten found improvements in strength and sensation that persisted for over one year. The largest trial (seventy patients) included people post-SCI by ten or more months with no recent neurologic improvement.[14] Among the fifty patients who received both rehabilitation therapy and transplantation of autologous BM-MSCs, nearly half had significant improvements in daily function, motor strength, and sensation, with no serious side effects, while the twenty control patients showed no change.

There have been forty-three completed clinical trials of stem cells, predominantly autologous BM-MSCs for the treatment of stroke.[15] The major difference from the SCI trials was that most patients were treated within seven days of their stroke. In the three largest trials completed, there were no significant benefits at three months.[16]

There have only been nine trials of stem cells for TBI, and only two of these have been completed.[17] The largest trial randomized forty patients with chronic TBI (>10 months post-injury) to MSCs derived from the umbilical cord compared to the usual treatment. There were statistically significant improvements of motor function in the upper and lower extremities, as well as sensation and balance.[18]

In summary, stem cell therapy for ANI remains at the earliest stages of development. Many important questions haven't yet been answered, including the type and dose of transplanted cells, best route of administration, timing relative to the initial injury, patient selection, biomarkers, effect of medications being taken as part of routine care (both positive and negative), and duration of benefit. The results of these trials are promising, but the degree of success has been limited. The good news is that none of these treatments has caused serious side effects. Unfortunately, though, none of the studies reported efficacy that would meet the standards required by the FDA for approval. You and your doctor should visit clinicaltrials.gov regularly to find trials that you may participate in, as well as the results of ongoing trials.

Drugs to Mobilize and Differentiate Stem Cells

While it's likely that different types of stem cells will be required to treat different ANIs, a common area of investigation will be the use of drugs to mobilize stem cells that are present in brain tissue. It has been well established that the brain's memory center (hippocampus), the smell center (olfactory nerve), and the ventricles of the brain contain stem cells. Our understanding of how to use drugs to differentiate these tissue stem cells into specific brain cell types (neurons, astrocytes, and glia) damaged by ANI is rapidly advancing.

Scaffolds and Drugs to Promote Nerve Regeneration

Improving regeneration of nerve tissues will require a multipronged approach. A key component is likely to be a scaffold that creates an environment favorable to regeneration. A more recent approach to regenerating nerves in people with SCI has been to combine stem cell transplantation with engineered scaffolds.[19] Scaffolds are made of proteins and other substances that together are called a "matrix," which has the consistency of gelatin. Some of the common matrix proteins are collagen, fibronectin, glucosamine, and chondroitin. These proteins assemble to form structures that look like scaffolds on buildings, which provide support and orientation to build and repair tissue. Several different types of scaffolds have been tested for nerve regeneration (most frequently in animals with SCI). These include scaffolds that contain enzymes that degrade scar tissue, release nerve growth factors, and provide shape and structure for the tissue. For treating SCI, these enzymes and growth factors are placed directly at the site of the SCI using nanoparticles or liposomes that release these factors in a slow, controlled manner over days to weeks. Finally, some specialized polymers may be injected to create 3D-scaffolds and tubes that enable the nerves to grow through the scar in the correct direction.

Neuroplasticity: Devices and Drugs

Through the concept of neuroplasticity, you can restore the function of your brain and body, bringing functionally dead parts of your nervous system back to life. Two key requirements for neuroplasticity are learning and practicing.

Computer-assisted learning: We all know that the more we practice a skill, the better we become at it. The same holds true for our senses, such as hearing, smelling, and seeing. If you had a TBI or stroke that caused you to experience vision loss, you would have to learn how to see again. I faced a similar problem learning how to hold a wine glass.

Learning often takes a lot of practice and repetition. But what if this learning process could be accelerated? For relearning vision, you need to know what to look for and how to consciously recognize the image your brain receives (perception). In one study, subjects performed a "motion threshold" task in which they learned how to detect motion of one marked object moving among many objects. They were then asked to perform the task while given different types of brain stimulation, each involving a non-invasive electrical current applied over the visual cortex. The researchers found that one type of brain stimulation, transcranial random noise stimulation (tRNS), had remarkable effects on improving the motion threshold.[20]

They extended their findings to patients who had suffered a stroke or TBI that made them partially blind. Combining tRNS brain stimulation with visual training therapy resulted in significant improvement in visual perception and function after only ten days.[21] More impressive, the improvement lasted more than six months, demonstrating permanent neurorestoration. It's possible that similar techniques can be used to improve other senses such as touch, temperature, taste, smell, and proprioception. Combining novel computer-based sensory training programs with tRNS represents a new approach to neurorestoration of human sensation, which represents an important advance in therapy.

Virtual reality: Virtual reality (VR) has been well studied in promoting the rehabilitation of motor, cognitive, and psychosocial functions in ANI patients, especially those with TBI.[22] VR has become cost-effective with improvements in head-mounted displays and hand controllers that can be purchased for $200 to $600. It's safe, though it may cause mild vertigo. VR offers the ability to simulate environments that foster neuroplasticity. It's particularly effective for complex functional actions, such as walking with a cane, reaching for and grabbing an object with one hand, or raising or lowering the object with two hands. Motions can be simulated with your hands each holding a controller that moves your avatar, a simulated figure of yourself. Repetitive trials using the avatar can be performed quickly, safely, and with no assistance to achieve the desired result. Because it's virtual, muscle fatigue is minimal and restarting the therapy takes no time or effort. Furthermore, VR can begin with easy tasks that become increasingly difficult on an individualized basis. This enables you to be successful at your appropriate level, and because success breeds success, the psychological aspects are positive rather than negative—especially important since many ANI patients have reactive depression. In addition, potentially dangerous or anxiety-provoking tasks, such as walking without handrails or a walker, can be performed without fear. To address the requirements of performing the activities of daily living, training multiple motor, sensory, and cognitive skills ("walking and chewing gum at the same time") is necessary. VR offers unique advantages to address this challenge because its interactive nature encourages training in an individualized manner. A clinical trial of VR in people with stroke and TBI showed that VR training improved performance not only in the trained task but also in specific neuropsychological functions such as visual memory retrieval. A review of studies that tested the effect of VR in people with TBI found that VR had the potential to be an effective assessment and rehabilitation tool for treatment of cognitive and behavioral impairment.[23] As computer and hardware technology improves, the use of VR in rehabilitation will likely be a major tool.

Enhancing Learning and Neuroplasticity

A fundamental concept for neurorestoration is learning how to perform old tasks using new nerves. Therefore, neuroplasticity must begin by understanding the mechanisms by which we learn: how memories are stored and then retrieved to perform learned tasks. This type of neuroplasticity requires that molecules be released from one nerve to the next to enable communication (hence the name, "neurotransmitters") between the parts of the brain that are responsible.

Molecules and proteins that stimulate neuroplasticity: Although many molecular signaling pathways are involved in learning and neuroplasticity, brain-derived neurotrophic factor (BDNF) has emerged as a prime facilitator of motor learning and rehabilitation after ANI.[24] Two strategies that have been shown to increase BDNF levels are aerobic exercise and certain neurotransmitters.[25] The therapeutic use of BDNF and these neurotransmitters has been shown in animals and will hopefully be tested in humans soon.[26]

Drugs: Accelerating learning and enhancing memory with drugs has enormous appeal for treatment of many neurological diseases. Drugs that promote neuroplasticity are called nootropics (from the Greek meaning "mind" and "a turning"), smart pills, or cognitive enhancers. Their benefits are measured by improved cognition, creativity, attention, memory, and decision-making. At this time, there are no FDA approved nootropics. However, there are many candidates[27]:

- The best cognitive enhancers are stimulants, like caffeine, and the prescription drugs dextroamphetamine and methylphenidate, which are used to treat attention deficit with hyperactivity disorder (ADHD). In particular, the classes of stimulants that demonstrate cognition-enhancing effects activate membrane proteins called receptors, especially the dopamine receptor D1 and adrenoceptor A2.[28]

- Donepezil is used to treat dementia in patients with Alzheimer's disease. It has been shown to improve memory, awareness, and the ability to function. It is an enzyme blocker that works by restoring the balance of endogenous neurotransmitters in the brain.[29]

- Selective serotonin reuptake inhibitors (SSRIs) have also shown promise. The first large-scale randomized clinical trial of SSRIs in acute stroke patients found that initiating the SSRI fluoxetine (Prozac) immediately after a stroke improved motor function at ninety days. This trial randomized half the patients to a placebo and half to fluoxetine, regardless of whether they had depression. Furthermore, an analysis of over four thousand stroke patients from multiple trials (including patients given SSRIs for depression) showed a similar benefit of SSRIs in recovery.[30]

Improving learning and memory with drugs alone has not been nearly as successful as using devices, but because there is such an enormous amount of research on people with dementia, it's likely that new drugs useful to people with ANI will also become available.

Integrative Medicine

Acupuncture

Traditional acupuncture involves needle insertion, moxibustion (burning dried mugwort on the skin over acupuncture meridians to improve circulation), and cupping therapy, as well as feeling the pulse for the strength and symmetry of your qi. Although many health providers think that acupuncture's benefits are due primarily to a placebo effect, recent studies in animals and people have identified a logical mechanism that has implications for new approaches to treating pain. Specifically, it was found that adenosine, a neuromodulator with pain-relieving properties, was released during acupuncture. Injection of a drug that activated the adenosine receptor also caused pain relief. With this knowledge, it should be possible to replicate the benefits of acupuncture using specific drugs, perhaps in combination with acupuncture needles.[31]

Probiotics

The communication between your gut microbiome (the bacteria that live in your intestines) and brain affects many aspects of brain function, including immune cell activation, formation of the blood-brain barrier, formation of new neurons, and myelination. Because the gut microbiome can be modified easily using antibiotics or probiotics, it represents a new target for drug development and for probiotic modulation. Several studies have shown effects of probiotics to alter the inflammatory response mediated by microglia and infiltrating macrophages, thereby protecting neurons from death. Future studies that identify beneficial molecules made by certain types of bacteria should provide new avenues for ANI therapies based on probiotics.[32]

Traditional Chinese Medicine (TCM)

TCM medications are currently not well understood in Western medicine. The variation among different manufacturers is so great that they are not safe to use. The Chinese government is spending more than $200 million each year to identify the molecules present in the medicines. I anticipate that new drugs will emerge from this intense research, some of which should be beneficial for people with ANI.

How to Participate in Clinical Trials

Progress in neurorestoration can only occur if clinical trials take place. There are many promising therapies on the horizon, so there should be opportunities for you to participate in a trial, if you so choose. There are three good reasons to volunteer for a clinical trial. First, you will be contributing to development of a possible new therapy for people like you. Second, you will receive high-quality clinical care that may improve your health in areas other than the objective of the trial. This care comes free of cost, and some trials may pay you for your participation. Third, you may benefit from a drug that you would not otherwise receive until FDA approval, which can take several years.

But there are a few caveats. It's possible that there may be unintended harmful side effects of the treatment. And participation in certain trials, especially those that require an intervention, may exclude you from future clinical trials. This is particularly likely if you receive stem cells or have a device implanted over your spinal cord or brain.

How to Find the Right Clinical Trial

Only participate in trials that have stringent safeguards. The trial's protocol should have undergone strict review by an Institutional Review Board (IRB), a standing committee of physicians, statisticians, community advocates, ethicists, and other experts who assess the risks and benefits to make the trial ethical and as safe as possible. They ensure that the participants are well informed and that their rights are protected. When you enroll, you should receive "informed consent" that describes the trial in as much detail as possible, especially the risks. You should never have to pay for a legitimate trial. Be extremely cautious about enrolling in a trial outside the United States, because not all countries have the same stringent reviews for safety.

You should believe in the potential benefit and significance of the therapy: There's nothing wrong with choosing a trial that may benefit you personally. But it's important to understand that the best trial designs include a placebo group. Neither you nor the investigators know who gets the therapy and who gets the placebo.

Your own doctors and family should support your decision: You should trust completely in the investigators who are leading the trial, and you should have the full support of your doctor and your family.

A Bright Future

Some of the devices, drugs, and other therapies discussed here may seem far-fetched. Certainly, a few years ago, some of them would have sounded like science fiction. But all of these things are real and hold great promise for neurorestoration after ANI. I have no doubt that some of the disabilities people live with after stroke, SCI, and TBI will be readily and effectively addressed with the therapies we see on the horizon. If you had told me about the iPad the month before my injury, I would have assumed that my ability to purchase one would be several years away. Yet it showed up only ten months after my injury. And as I look into the future, I'm confident that the inventiveness of the human mind and our unquenchable thirst to discover and create will bring many new treatments that make our lives even better.

The Power of Hope and Love

Leading a Life that Continues to Astound Me

> *You may not control all the events that happen to you,*
> *but you can decide not to be reduced by them.*

> —Maya Angelou

As I write this, almost twelve years have passed since my injury. (But who's counting?) No matter how much time goes by, I remember the event vividly. When I was transported by helicopter to the emergency room, all I hoped for was to live. I knew I had suffered a serious injury and that my recovery, if any, would be a long, difficult journey. In retrospect, it has been more difficult and much longer than I imagined.

While I sensed I would be able to keep parts of my old life, I learned I would also have to let some things go. And I would have to be open to incorporating the "new"—new skills, new habits, and new people. What I didn't understand until later was that, to be happy again, I would have to build a new life. I've now done that, and it's a life that continues to astound me. My home and family life, friendships, social activities, professional work, and community involvement—all of them are rich and full and bring me more joy than I ever envisioned.

At the time of my injury, I was living the dream—I'd achieved tremendous success in my work as a physician and researcher, father to three wonderful adult children, and living in a place and manner I had aspired to since I was in college. At work, I had advanced to CEO of the University of Rochester Medical Center. Life was good. But a bicycle accident turned all that on its head.

One year after my accident, thanks to the compassion of my colleagues at the University of Rochester, I was able to return to my prior role. I am forever grateful to them for that opportunity. Being able to work, even on a part-time basis, helped me persevere through the hard days of rehabilitation, and enabled me to believe that I *could* have a future that included meaningful employment—and a way to support myself and my family.

A lot has happened between then and now. My first marriage eventually ended in divorce, unable to withstand the strain of my new situation. I've learned more about wheelchairs, various catheters, urine bags, neuropathic pain, swallowing, and rehabilitation than I ever cared to. I've made new friends; remarried; had four more grandchildren; lost my mother; and changed who I was, to become who I am. And I'm a better person because of everything I've experienced and, more important, everyone I've met.

Today, I'm the director of the University of Rochester Neurorestoration Institute (URNI), where our motto is "using the mind to restore the brain and body." The people who come to us have suffered an acute neurological injury, like I have, and are looking for new ways to improve their quality of life. Our mission is "to restore functions lost or impaired by damage to the brain and spinal cord." It's the most rewarding endeavor of my medical career. Every day, my colleagues and I are working hard to make the URNI a nationally recognized leader in rehabilitation and restoration of cognitive, motor, and sensory function.

Has getting here been easy? In a word: no. Worth the effort? Oh, yes.

For one thing, my time as a patient changed me as a doctor. It expanded my understanding of the need for more attentiveness, compassion, teamwork, and respectful two-way communication by health care providers with the patient and family. The insights I gained during my time in the hospital, and since then, have become the philosophy that guides every member of the health care team at the URNI.

I also became a more outgoing person. Now, when I wheel through the hospital on my way to physical therapy, I say hello to everyone I see (and I make an effort to learn everyone's names), from the CEO to volunteers to environmental services workers. Without fail, this simple interaction brings a smile to all parties.

I got over my hang-up about never needing help. Learning to acknowledge that I do need assistance at times has made me a humbler person. And it has forced me to slow down a bit, which has reminded me of the importance of always using the word *please*. And saying *thank you*. I've learned that most people are generous and, when given the opportunity, want to help. These connections with others are mutually beneficial, feeding our souls and making our days on this earth more meaningful.

There has been a lot of hard mental, physical, and emotional work to get to where I am today, and I still face challenges. Sometimes, the past intrudes on the present, when I realize how much I've lost—a relationship severed because I didn't fully appreciate the effort the person was making, or an activity like hiking, which will be forever lost. When I find myself looking backward, I lean on my mantra: *Forgive, let it go, move on.* It helps.

I've forged new relationships with my children. At the time of my accident, my kids were thirty-two, twenty-six, and twenty-three. They were all living independently and had established their own lives. Over the past twelve years, we've redefined our connections and are actually much closer now than we were before my injury. I think my accident revealed the fragility of life; that, plus the pain the divorce caused them, made each of us aware how important our family is. These realizations have helped us establish stronger bonds and have given us the ability to have more honest conversations.

When my former wife and I separated, I was quite lonely. I made an effort to reconnect with friends whom, previously, I would see only once in a great while. Getting together to watch sports on TV or go to a baseball game was an excellent starting point. Baseball was particularly good because I could bring my grandchildren with me (for the food, not the game!).

I dearly missed biking, despite the fact that I had been on my bike when I had my accident. Eventually, I bought a three-wheeled recumbent bike (Figure 33) and invited a few friends to ride with me on the weekends. Soon, there were four or five of us riding every weekend. I then graduated to a faster, safer tricycle and began riding the roads. Today, I ride my recumbent three-wheeler every Thursday and Sunday—with friends—all year, except for the winter months. I even participate in longer charity rides (15–25 miles/24–40 km), when the opportunity arises. The friendships that have come from this shared passion for biking have made my life fuller and given me more to look forward to.

Among my new friends are the Push Men, all SCI paraplegics and tetraplegics who have spent twenty-five years or more in wheelchairs. We get together every two to three months for dinner, and in between those gatherings, we're there to help one another out with any kind of problem. They've helped me tremendously over the years because each one of them has intimate knowledge of almost every problem I face.

Getting divorced and being single again after more than thirty years of marriage was a big transition. I settled into bachelorhood with dinner parties and sports activities. But I was lonely for a close companion, a woman with whom I could enjoy life. I missed romance and intimacy. After a year on my own, I began to let friends know I was open to dating, hoping that those couples who knew me well would magically find the perfect blind date. Unfortunately, my brilliant plan only revealed that our tastes in women were vastly different.

But, eventually, I met a woman whose smile just made me feel good. It was near Christmas and I wanted to enjoy a fun meal, so I called her up to ask her to dine with me. She later told me that she spent three hours deciding whether to say yes. We're both glad that she did, and we've been together ever since.

Since my injury in 2009, I've often heard a voice in my head saying, *You can accomplish anything as long as you set your mind to do it.* My mother told me this many times as I was growing up, but never was it more helpful than during rehabilitation. The memory of her words reminds me that it's my responsibility to lead a good life, and there's nothing to gain from blaming those around me. There certainly are occasions when frustration at my circumstances sets in. It's not fun when I go through a period of bladder spasms and leak urine around my suprapubic tube—it's an obvious reminder that my life has changed dramatically.

In October 2017, I traveled to Nanjing, China, to spend six weeks at Zhongshan Rehabilitation Hospital. The time I spent in Zhongshan Hospital was eye-opening—I learned firsthand about the benefits of traditional Chinese medicine (TCM). In particular, I discovered that acupuncture, massage, and meditation had dramatic beneficial effects on my physical and mental health. And, over the next six months, I was able to reduce my neuropathic pain medications such as pregabalin (Lyrica) from 400 mg to 50 mg per day. I quickly reduced my other pain and spasticity medications as well, changing to a combination of Tylenol and nortriptyline, and reducing baclofen from 130 mg to 70 mg per day. My daytime drowsiness disappeared almost completely.

It wasn't only the rehab and medications in China that were having such dramatic effects on my function, but also the change in what I was eating. In China, we ate a mostly plant-based diet—we rarely ate meat, although we did eat fish and other seafood regularly. There were no processed carbohydrates like bread, cookies, or pasta. This is the diet I follow now, and I'm convinced it has helped my gut health, which science shows is integral to brain health.

My immersion in Chinese rehabilitation and lifestyle provided the perfect opportunity for me to practice mindfulness, meditation, and self-awareness. I believe that my improved self-image was the most important psychological change that occurred in China. This empowered me to focus on my most important long-term goals and what I needed to do to achieve them.

But the most important rehabilitation lesson I learned from my time in China was the value of walking. During the first year after my accident, I had learned to walk up to seventy-five feet using a platform walker (Figure 32, see page 209). But this talent had no benefit on my daily life, because I could only go a short distance before my shoulders started to hurt. I decided it was a better use of my time to work on my upper body strength and function, since it would enable me to be more independent when eating and using my computer, for example. Even the therapeutic approaches that emphasized intense treadmill walking in a harness seemed like a waste of time, because this training doesn't enable you to walk safely outside of the treadmill on flat surfaces like wood and linoleum. But what I learned in China was that *walking can improve your sensory and autonomic nervous system function*. This was a huge revelation. And I came to believe that the mind-brain-body system can work in reverse: changes in the body can be transmitted upward to improve the functions of the brain and mind.

In China, I learned to walk using my platform walker again. I now walk five days a week and have gradually increased my time to fifteen minutes each day. I've also dramatically increased the speed of my walking; it's now more than twice as fast as it was in 2017. The benefits to my overall health have been phenomenal—increased bone density, better bowel function, more muscle mass, and cardiovascular improvements. For someone who spends most of the day in a wheelchair, the psychological benefit of standing and walking cannot be overstated.

When I returned to work in 2010 as CEO of the University of Rochester Medical Center, I knew that, eventually, I wanted to go in a new direction: one that would help people like me. But first I needed to complete a major project—financing and building a new children's hospital—which took five years. When that project was completed, in 2015, I turned my focus to the development of a multidisciplinary clinical center for people with ANI—the University of Rochester Neurorestoration Institute (URNI), where I now serve as director. I considered the establishment of the URNI a necessity; there was no place in western New York that patients with ANI could go for comprehensive evaluation of all neurological and medical issues, treatment recommendations, and participation in clinical trials.

Several studies were published at that time about the use of devices to treat neurologic diseases, especially ANI. These reports reminded me of the late 1980s in cardiology, when there was an explosion of devices (pacemakers, implantable defibrillators, balloon angioplasty, and coronary artery stents). These devices transformed the practice of cardiology. I saw remarkable parallels in neurorehabilitation and wanted to be part of it.

In addition to bringing specialists together to evaluate and recommend therapies, the URNI will recruit people to participate in multicenter clinical trials. The medical specialties will include internal medicine, cardiology, neurology, physiatry, orthopedics, urology, and mental health. There will also be other professionals available to consult with patients and their families on nutrition, equipment, financial aid, and support groups. After a patient receives a complete evaluation, a physiatrist will assemble all of the necessary information and provide recommendations for medications, rehabilitation, nutrition, and possible clinical trials.

I'm honored to say that I have collaborated with two superb researchers— Jon Wolpaw, MD (director, National Center for Adaptive Neurotechnologies) and Rajiv Ratan, MD, PhD (executive director of the Burke Neurological Institute)—to create a new clinical research program for people with ANI called NeuroCuresNY. The first clinical trial will begin in September 2021. We hope that our research network will ultimately become a magnet for people with ANI who want to participate in clinical trials of new devices and new drugs.

After people in my community told me I inspired them, I began making that role part of my mission. Having accepted the challenge to be an inspiration, I've used my position in health care to advocate for improved accessibility in local organizations, and especially at not-for-profit entities. At the state level, I've continued to participate in the funding committee of the New York State Stem Cell Science program (NYSTEM), which funds meritorious research in stem cell approaches, including nerve regeneration in several neurological diseases. I've also supported funding for the New York State Spinal Cord Injury Research Board (SCIRB). Recently, I received funding for my first project on improving spinal cord function using drugs that decrease inflammation. These efforts are part of my "pay it forward" pledge to help others.

I'm confident that five years from now I will have dramatically increased my independence with new devices. I'm fairly confident that there will be an SCS device that can relieve the pain in my right arm and ameliorate my complex regional pain syndrome. I also think that, with epidural electrical stimulation, there's a good chance I'll be able to walk longer and, I hope, with only minimal support (using a walker or cane). I'm less confident but still hopeful that more walking will improve my bladder, bowel, and sexual function. I'm also hopeful that I'll be able to purchase a self-driving vehicle that can take me safely wherever I want to go.

As I finish writing this book, we are in the midst of the COVID-19 pandemic, and I have been self-isolated for months. Everyone is talking about an indefinite "new normal" of wearing masks, practicing social distancing, and washing our hands repeatedly throughout the day. But there's no way this scenario is normal. Nor should you see your life immediately after your injury as your "new normal." Yes, you are on a new and unanticipated path, but I want you to view it as the start of a new life in which you can experience an ongoing recovery.

When I lay on the ground with a broken neck in 2009, praying I would live to see my family one more time, I couldn't have envisioned the life I lead today. My wife and I take international vacations, I'm active in local civic events, and I'm an advocate for people with disabilities on a local and state level. After my injury, I had to relearn to swallow; once I could do that safely, I was spoon-fed by an aide because my arms were too weak. Now, I can feed myself, hold a wine glass, and even pour wine for my wife.

I've gotten here with two elixirs available to each of us: hope and love. Hope provides the motivation to work hard on rehabilitation. Love provides the emotional support it takes to overcome the hurdles. I have no doubt that I will continue to recover even more function in the days, months, and years ahead. And you will, too. Whatever stage of rehab you're at, know that you can and will achieve even more. An astounding future awaits you. As you make your way on this journey, I send you love, encouragement, and hope.

Keep me posted. I'd love to hear from you at drbradberk.com.

Brad Berk, MD, PhD
2021

Acknowledgments

. book, like most projects, is a team effort. I was very fortunate to have an excellent team who have worked tirelessly to help me physically, mentally, and emotionally, to maintain my dedication and determination to finish this book. It has taken five long years from start to finish, and I have many people to thank for helping me cross the finish line.

First, the beginning. While I was lying in the ICU, unable to move or talk, I had plenty of time to think. I developed the framework for a book that would be one part autobiography, one part medicine, and one part guide to the mental and emotional challenges that you face recovering from a severe neurological injury. Three years later, I had the time, energy and enthusiasm to begin writing. I discussed my ideas with my therapist, Alice Rubenstein, who connected me with Dr. Julie Silver, a rehab specialist and researcher who taught in the *Writing, Publishing, and Social Media for Healthcare Professionals* course at Harvard Medical School. I emailed her with my idea and asked if she would discuss it with me. To my surprise, she answered immediately and positively. But, when I finished presenting my three-part idea, she told me that I had committed every sin a first-time writer could commit. She then advised me to write a self-help book instead. And so my journey began.

My family has been the bedrock of my recovery and has provided input into the book at every stage. My wife, Dr. Coral Surgeon, has been the sounding board for every chapter that stymied me. More importantly, she has provided a female perspective and has epitomized the fine line between caregiver and spouse. I cannot thank her enough for her expertise in both roles. My children and grandchildren have provided me with boundless moments of joy. When my accident happened, I had three grandsons. I now have seven grandchildren who have all taken joyrides in "Poppa's" wheelchair.

Mariah, my older daughter, opened a CaringBridge site where friends, colleagues, and other people in the community could send me their notes of encouragement, support, and positive thinking. Her husband, Anthony, was a morning fixture when I was in the ICU at Strong Memorial Hospital. He would bring his cup of coffee and the morning newspaper to read stories to me. It was great to have a touch of normalcy in the ICU. My son, Dave, was one of the primary reasons I went to Kessler Rehabilitation Institute, because he lived only twenty-five minutes away. We had a Wednesday night date for dinner that he always made, where we could discuss politics, finance, and my recovery (in that order). We spent more time together in my one hundred days at Kessler than in the many years before my accident, and it was wonderful to learn more about each other.

My younger daughter, Sarah, was working for the US State Department, traveling the world and providing community health programs on preventing maternal-to-fetal AIDS transmission. She always sent me funny emails from wherever she had landed and amazed me with her boundless enthusiasm for a very difficult project. My sister, Karen, and her husband, Allan, have been there whenever I needed them. Mercifully, it has usually been for positive events, such as bicycling or holidays all year round.

I also have to thank my mother, who didn't change one bit after my accident. Her one comment about my injury was, "Brad, you've always been able to achieve what you wanted when you had the determination to get there." Sadly, she died in 2012, but she still observed an enormous improvement in my abilities. My ex-wife, Mary, took on the incredibly challenging task of transitioning us to a lifestyle that imposed few limits and afforded each of us freedom and independence, from one that was filled with hardship and limitations.

I've been fortunate to have met many wonderful people in my time in Rochester. Mark and Lois Taubman have been close friends since he and I were in training for cardiology in the 1980s, and our children grew up together. He came to Rochester in 2003, and from May 2009 to May 2010 he served as the CEO of URMC while I was in the hospital and during my recovery. Mark and Lois are our closest friends, and their encouragement and joy in my recovery has been heartwarming. Laurie Kopin was my clinical cardiology nurse until my accident. Since then, she has assisted me many times when I have been asked by friends and fellow ANI patients to help with their care. David and Dawn Klein have been close friends in business and pleasure. When David and I traveled to France on a wine tour in 2011, his compassion, attentiveness, and help made it a wonderful adventure. Tim Doherty has been a family friend since his son Robert grew up with my daughter Mariah. Always calling me "Berky," he has challenged me many times to "do more," and has been there to do more himself. He was instrumental in forming my cycling group, A Krew of Pirates (our motto is "we travel to the west and take no prisoners"). The rest of the Krew—Johnny Fahner-Vihtelic, Peter Keenan, Harvey Botzman, and Mike Schell—have made every ride a laugh a minute.

Thank you to my other group of buddies, the Push Men—Rob Tortorella, Bill Sykes, Bob Morgan, and Dave Hebert. We help each other with every problem that someone with a SCI encounters. My skiing partner, Jason Swinton, not only keeps me safe on the slopes but also makes the best sausage I have ever tasted. Thank you also to Rick Aab and Tami Wihlen, Mike and Alice Smith, Rob Callihan and Nana Bennett, Jim and Judy Fonzi, John and Cindy LiDestri, Karen and Larry Kessler, Travis and Katie Betters, and Sherwood Deutsch.

I'm very fortunate to work with a fantastic group of physicians and psychologists who are not only superb clinicians but also caring and compassionate individuals. Thank you to Steve Kirshblum, Kanakadurga (Durgi) Poduri, Dick Burton, Rich Barbano, David Dobrinzki, Jean Nickels, Chuck Wadsworth, Gareth Warren, Alice Rubinstein, and Jeff Levenkron.

My occupational and physical therapists have continued to work with me over the last eleven years to help me prove that continuous therapy results in steady improvement. Tim O'Connor, Cindy Thielman, Kathy Owens, and Simon Carson have shown me numerous ways to achieve my goals of greater independence.

I have been helped by terrific assistants and aides over the last eleven years. My first assistant, Harley Bowman, originally trained as a safety officer to help local companies prepare for OSHA inspections. Harley impressed me with his safety-first approach, infinite patience, and compassion. He picked me up every morning and drove me to work. He made me lunch, helped me get from one appointment to another, helped me stretch, and assisted me through the day so that I wouldn't be too tired to be a good husband when I got home. After seven years, when Harley retired, I was very fortunate to find a new assistant, Sean Hopkins, who has stepped into Harley's big shoes with no problem. The only significant difference between Sean and Harley is that Sean is young enough to be one of my children, and he is incredibly strong, which makes everything effortless.

Thank you also to Barbara Conti Anderson and Sharon Steele-Jones, who contributed enormously to my initial recovery and progress. Barbara was an amazing combination of aide, assistant, design artist, clothes specialist, and organizer. She took charge of everything in my life except for personal grooming and showers, which were Sharon's expertise. Sharon learned my morning and evening programs at Strong Memorial Hospital and was my morning aide for over six years. It was wonderful sharing news about our family and friends each morning. Catherine (Cat) Williams was a live-in aide for one year. She accompanied us on several trips and helped us with cooking, cleaning, and my personal care.

Thank you to Susan Merkel, Dan Andrus, Judy Halling, Emily Halling, Joella Ellingwood, Laura Rasmussen, Hannah Santini, Autumn Wenzel, Bonny Waden, Kristin Terranova, Julian Goodsell, Akila Fenton, Dajanique Montgomery, and Cassie Flamm, all dedicated personal aides.

I've also been fortunate to have a series of secretaries/administrators who have managed my work and home schedules, helped me pay the bills, and filled in whenever Sean was unavailable. Joyce Goodberlet was my secretary/administrator from 2001 until I stepped down in 2015. She was unflappable, an excellent editor, and a calming influence. Ellen Caruso, who has remained a close personal contact, worked with me for six months as I transitioned back to CEO full time. In my new role as the director of the URNI, I have had a string of wonderful secretaries/administrators, including Bradley Hamling, Heather Salatino, Pat Zubil, David Merulla, and now Jennifer Rosenzweig.

Professionally, I've been helped by many former postdoctoral fellows in the lab who have gone on to pursue independent careers. The Yin family—Guoyong and his wife, Yingqian Xu, and daughter Shiqian—have become close colleagues and friends. They hosted me in Nanjing twice and introduced me to Dr. Jianan Li, who has made an enormous difference in my rehabilitation. Other students who have become faculty include Jun-ichi Abe, Zheng-Gen Jin, Slava Korshunov, Stefanie Lehoux, Jinjiang Pang, and Chen Yan. They have matured into wonderful colleagues who have helped me and collaborated with me over the last eleven years.

I owe a great deal to my postdoctoral fellows, several of whom carried on independently while I was in the hospital and in recovery: Sayantani Chowdhury, Chia Hsu, Syamantak Majumder, Himanshu Meghwani, Megan Cavet, Patty Nigro, Kimio Satoh, Nwe Nwe Soe, Shin-Young Park, Elaine Smolock, Lian Wang, and Cameron World.

I've also been blessed with terrific graduate students, including Lingli Li, Naoya Maekawa, Marlene Mathews, Prashanthi Menon, Xi Shi, Oded Spindel, Xiao-Qun Wang, and Chao Xue. Two long-term members of my lab group, Mark Sowden and Mary Wines-Samuelson, both research scientists, have contributed their superb knowledge of molecular biology and biochemistry as well as their love of teaching and warm hearts to the fellows, graduate students, and me.

I am deeply indebted to Joel Seligman (former president of the University of Rochester) and Ed Hajim (former chairman of the Board of Trustees at UR), for their confidence in me. They could not have known how much recovery I would achieve and how capable I would be of handling the mental and physical stress of being CEO. They waited one year to see the results, and I know that I repaid them for their belief. It is rare to have two bosses with such faith.

This book could not have been written without the assistance of three special people. I was so lucky to have Martha Murphy as my cowriter. I very much appreciate her insights into health care. Martha helped me write a book proposal, which led to Linda Konner's becoming my agent. With her help, we found Olivia Peluso as my editor and The Experiment as my publisher. Linda and Olivia have been brilliant in making the book better organized. In particular, I want to thank Olivia for rethinking the book's structure and helping me shorten it to a half-day read. In addition, a special thanks to Michal Shaposhnikov for creating and adapting many figures, and to Shehanez Ellika for providing CT scans.

Finally, I'd like to thank Dr. Jianan Li. I met Dr. Li shortly after my accident through Dr. Guoyong Yin. I met Dr. Li on my first visit to China after my accident. He gave me a tour of the new campus for Zhongshan

Hospital and described his vision for a multidisciplinary center for SCI and TBI, very similar to the URNI. He convinced me that a sustained program of walking would have enormous benefits for my autonomic nervous system, especially my bowel and bladder. So one crazy day in October 2016, Coral, Sean Hopkins, and I flew to China. The day after arriving, I began six hours of therapy daily, and weekly meetings with Dr. Li to optimize my rehab program. Dr. Li was inspirational in his belief that "man was meant to walk," so walking farther, faster, and more often should improve my autonomic nervous system and sensorimotor function. Within two weeks, I noticed improvements in my complex regional pain syndrome (less pain, more blood flow) and sensorimotor function (I could feel my right leg better). After six weeks, I could walk twice as far and 50 percent faster. This personal breakthrough convinced me to seek further treatments to improve walking. My next "step" will be to enroll in a clinical trial of EES or transcutaneous ES to achieve independent walking. I am confident that with the support of the many people who have already helped me, I will succeed.

In closing, I want to thank you for reading my book. Whether you are someone with an ANI, a family member, caregiver, or friend, I know that you are searching for ways to improve recovery. I hope this book empowers you to keep working to get better, and that it serves as a source of motivation, determination, and resilence. As you travel the long road to recovery, live each day to the fullest, and remember to thank those around you for their help.

Resources

General Resources for All ANIs

Books

Gary Karp. *Life on Wheels: The A to Z Guide to Living Fully with Mobility Issues*, second edition. New York: Demos Health, 2008.

Norman Doidge, MD. *The Brain That Changes Itself: Stories of Personal Triumph from the Frontiers of Brain Science*, reprint edition. New York: Penguin, 2007.

Norman Doidge, MD. *The Brain's Way of Healing: Remarkable Discoveries and Recoveries from the Frontiers of Neuroplasticity*, updated edition. New York: Penguin, 2016.

Websites

- Americans with Disability Act: ada.gov
- Centers for Disease Control and Prevention (CDC): cdc.gov
- Clinical trials: clinicaltrials.gov
- Mayo Clinic: mayoclinic.org
- National Institutes of Health: nih.gov
- National Heart, Lung, and Blood Institute (NHLBI): nhlbi.nih.gov
- National Institute on Disability, Independent Living, and Rehabilitation Research (NIDILRR): acl.gov
- National Institute of Mental Health (NIMH): nimh.nih.gov
- National Institute for Neurologic Disorders and Stroke (NINDS): ninds.nih.gov

- National Center for Complementary and Integrative Health (NCCIH): nccih.nih.gov
- Christopher and Dana Reeve Foundation: christopherreeve.org/living-with-paralysis/free-resources-and-downloads/paralysis-resource-guide
- UpToDate: uptodate.com
- US Department of Veterans Affairs: Office of Research and Development: research.va.gov

Books and Websites on Specific Topics

- Advocacy
  - Americans Disabled for Attendant Programs Today (ADAPT), a national grassroots community that works to assure the civil and human rights of people with disabilities: adapt.org
  - American Association of People with Disabilities (AAPD), a national voice for change in implementing the goals of the ADA: aapd.com
  - Patient Advocate Foundation (PAF): patientadvocate.org

- Diets, Eating Plans, Nutrition, RDAs:
  - nhlbi.nih.gov/health-topics/dash-eating-plan
  - heart.org/en/healthy-living/healthy-eating/eat-smart/nutrition-basics/mediterranean-diet
  - canada.ca/en/health-canada/services/food-nutrition/healthy-eating/dietary-reference-intakes/consumer-guide-dris-dietary-reference-intakes.html; obtain a PDF of *A Consumer's Guide to the DRIs (Dietary Reference Intakes)*
  - Michael Greger, MD. *How Not to Die: Discover the Foods Scientifically Proven to Prevent and Reverse Disease.* New York: Flatiron Books, 2015.
  - Jason Fung, MD. *The Obesity Code: Unlocking the Secrets of Weight Loss.* Vancouver, BC: Greystone Books, 2016.
  - Dorothy Calimeris and Lulu Cook, RDN. *The Complete Anti-Inflammatory Diet for Beginners.* Emeryville, CA: Rockridge Press, 2017.
  - Thomas Campbell, MD. *The China Study Solution: The Simple Way to Lose Weight and Reverse Illness, Using a Whole-Food, Plant-Based Diet.* Emmaus, PA: Rodale, 2016.

- Disability Products & Services
  - Amazon has the most comprehensive site for disability products in its health section. I purchase all of my disposable medical and supplies (e.g., pads, OTC supplements, vitamin C, melatonin, Tylenol, gloves, and so on) via amazon.com.

- United Spinal Association Disability Products & Services Directory: askus-resource-center.unitedspinal.org/index.php?pg=kb.page&id=3168
- Assistive Technology Industry Association: atia.org/home/at-resources
- Accessible and inclusive fashion:
  - kizik.com (hands-free sneakers)
  - seasaltcornwall.co.uk/clothing/easy-on-adaptive-clothing
- Employment Resources, Disability Rights, and Work Incentives
  - Department of Vocational Rehabilitation in your state is usually the best site to find programs that you are qualified to participate.
  - Rehabilitation Services Administration is part of the US Department of Education: rsa.ed.gov/about/programs. It has many programs to assist people with disabilities, including disability employment programs that work with state vocational rehabilitation services and state supported employment services.
  - Programs that protect you from discrimination in the workplace include
    - United States Equal Employment Opportunity Commission: eeoc.gov
    - Disability and Business Technical Assistance Centers. There are ten regional centers supported as part of the ADA National Network, adata.org, funded by the National Institute on Disability, Independent Living, and Rehabilitation Research (NIDILRR). The centers promote voluntary compliance with the Americans with Disabilities Act (ADA) by providing three core services: technical assistance, training, and materials dissemination.
    - Fair Employment Practice Agency (FEPA). Many states, counties, cities, and towns have their own laws prohibiting discrimination, as well as Fair Employment Practices Agencies (FEPAs) responsible for enforcing those laws. Usually the laws enforced by these agencies are similar to those enforced by EEOC: eeoc.gov/fair-employment-practices-agencies-fepas-and-dual-filing.
    - Ticket to Work and Work Incentives Improvement Act is a federally funded employment program designed to provide Social Security disability beneficiaries (i.e., individuals receiving SSDI and/or SSI benefits based on disability) the choices, opportunities, and support they need to enter the workforce and maintain employment with the goal of becoming economically self-supporting over time: yourtickettowork.ssa.gov/index.html.

- Exercise plans
  - Workout videos (also free) on YouTube and through online search for "wheelchair workouts"
  - themiamiproject.org/wp-content/uploads/2015/07/home-strength-training-guide-paraplegia.pdf
  - newmobility.com/2020/04/stay-at-home-wheelchair-workouts
- Health insurance and Financial support
  - Social Security Administration's Plan to Achieve Self-Support (PASS): ssa.gov/disabilityresearch/wi/pass.htm
  - Social Security Disability Income (SSDI): ssa.gov/benefits/disability
  - Supplemental Security Income (SSI): ssa.gov/benefits/ssi
- Medications
  - Patient Advocate Foundation is a national organization that can help you negotiate bills with hospitals, doctors, and insurance companies: patientadvocate.org.
  - Partnership for Prescription Assistance is a clearinghouse for more than 475 public and private assistance programs; it includes nearly 200 pharmaceutical options: screening.mhanational.org/content/partnership-prescription-assistance.
  - RxAssist: rxassist.org
  - NeedyMeds: needymeds.org
- The Resilience Project: theresilienceproject.com.au/about
- Travel and vacation service providers
  - Tour guides that focus on disability clients
    - disneyworld.disney.go.com/guest-services/guests-with-disabilities
    - disneycruise.disney.go.com/port-adventures/new-port-adventures-accessible-travel-solutions
    - executiveclasstravelers.com/1/travel_agents.htm
  - Air Ambulances
    - Angel Medflight: angelmedflight.com
    - Use your local not-for-profit air ambulance service, as their cost will be much lower than the for-profit national chains.
  - Renting places to stay
    - Airbnb: airbnb.com
    - VRBO: vrbo.com/vacation-rentals
  - Comparing credit cards for travel benefits
    - nerdwallet.com
    - wallethub.com

Resources for SCI

Books

Mayo Clinic Guide to Living with a Spinal Cord Injury: Moving Ahead with Your Life by Mayo Clinic

Spinal Cord Injury: A Guide for Living Second Edition, by Sara Palmer, PhD, Kay Harris Kriegsman, PhD, and Jeffrey B. Palmer, MD

Spinal Cord Medicine: Comprehensive Evidence-Based Clinical Reference for Diagnosis and Treatment of Spinal Cord Injuries and Conditions by Steven Kirshblum, MD, and Vernon W. Lin, PhD

Websites

- Paralyzed Veterans of America: pva.org
- United Spinal Association: unitedspinal.org
- Miami Project to Cure Paralysis: themiamiproject.org
- Abilities Not Disabilities!: facebook.com/groups/1524512594326787
- SCI Survivors: facebook.com/groups/Strokesupportgroup1
- Spinal Cord Journal and International Spinal Cord Society: facebook.com/groups/102413657179114
- Spinal Cord Injury USA Group: facebook.com/groups/2014869075503756
- Wives and Girlfriends of Spinal Cord Injury: wagsofsci.com
- WheelChair Mafia: facebook.com/WheelchairmafiaNL

Resources for Stroke

- American Stroke Association and American Heart Association: strokeassociation.org
- Stroke Survivors: facebook.com/groups/573759576077398
- Life After Stroke: facebook.com/groups/598682020276507
- Stroke Recovery Support Group: facebook.com/groups/1989966117920808
- Centers for Disease Control and Prevention: cdc.gov/stroke

Resources for TBI

Books

John W. Cassidy, MD. *Mindstorms: The Complete Guide for Families Living with Traumatic Brain Injury*. New York: Da Capo Lifelong Books, 2009.

Vani Rao, MBBS, MD, and Sandeep Vaishnavi, MD, PhD. *The Traumatized Brain: A Family Guide to Understanding Mood, Memory, and Behavior after Brain Injury*. Baltimore: Johns Hopkins University Press.

Amy Newmark and Dr. Carolyn Roy-Bornstein. *Chicken Soup for the Soul: Recovering from Traumatic Brain Injuries: 101 Stories of Hope, Healing, and Hard Work*. Chicken Soup for the Soul Publishing, 2014.

Dr. Dan Engle. *The Concussion Repair Manual: A Practical Guide to Recovering from Traumatic Brain Injuries*. Lifestyle Entrepreneurs Press, 2017.

Websites

TBI

- Brain Injury Association of America: biausa.org/public-affairs/media?search=%22concussion+information+center%22
- TraumaticBrainInjury.com: traumaticbraininjury.com
- Love Your Brain: facebook.com/loveyourbrainfoundation
- Traumatic or Acquired Brain Injury Support Group: facebook.com/groups/6367734334
- The Centers for Disease Control and Prevention: HEADS UP on Brain Injury Basics includes how to diagnose a concussion and specific recommendations for return to school and return to sports: cdc.gov/headsup/basics/index.html
- Traumatic Brain Injury Support Group: facebook.com/Traumatic-Brain-Injury-Support-Group-180684948672011
- TBI Hope & Inspiration: facebook.com/tbihopeandinspiration
- Traumatic Brain Injury Healing and Recovering Support Group: facebook.com/groups/186712754690242
- Traumatic Brain Injury Awareness and Support: facebook.com/groups/traumaticbraininjuryawareness

Notes

Introduction

David S. Goldstein, *Principles of Autonomic Medicine*, vol. 4, 2017. Accessed at: dir.ninds.nih.gov/publications/PrinciplesofAutonomicMedicinev40.pdf.

Chapter 1

1. American Psychological Association, "Cognitive behavior therapy." Accessed at dictionary.apa.org/cognitive-behavior-therapy.
2. American Psychiatric Association, *The Practice of Electroconvulsive Therapy: Recommendations for Treatment, Training, and Privileging*, 2nd ed. Washington, DC: American Psychiatric Publishing, 2001.
   Marcelo T. Berlim, et al., "Clinically meaningful efficacy and acceptability of low-frequency repetitive transcranial magnetic stimulation (rTMS) for treating primary major depression: A meta-analysis of randomized, double-blind and sham-controlled trials," *Neuropsychopharmacology* 38, no. 4 (November 2012): 543–51.
3. Stephanie Jarvi Steele, et al., "Efficacy of the Unified Protocol for transdiagnostic treatment of comorbid psychopathology accompanying emotional disorders compared to treatments targeting single disorders," Journal of Psychiatric Research 104 (September 2018): 211–16.
4. American Stroke Association, "Identifying and Treating Post-Stroke Depression Audiocast," September 6, 2019. Accessed at stroke.org/en/professionals/stroke-resource-library/adult-stroke-rehabilitation-and-recovery-audiocast-series/identifying-and-treating-post-stroke-depression.
5. O. Köhler, et al., "Effect of anti-inflammatory treatment on depression, depressive symptoms, and adverse effects: A systematic review and meta-analysis of randomized clinical trials," *JAMA Psychiatry* 71, no. 12 (December 2014): 1381–91.
6. J. P. Lefaucheur, et al., "Evidence-based guidelines on the therapeutic use of repetitive transcranial magnetic stimulation (rTMS)," *Clinical Neurophysiology* 125, no. 11 (November 2014): 2150–206.
7. American Heart Association, "How Does Depression Affect the Heart?" Accessed at heart.org/en/healthy-living/healthy-lifestyle/mental-health-and-wellbeing/how-does-depression-affect-the-heart.
8. American Psychiatric Association, *Diagnostic and Statistical Manual of Mental Disorders*, 5th ed. Arlington, VA: American Psychiatric Publishing, 2013.

9. L. Borza, "Cognitive-behavioral therapy for generalized anxiety," *Dialogues in Clinical Neuroscience* 19, no. 2 (June 2017): 203–8.
10. B. E. Cohen, et al., "State of the art review: Depression, stress, anxiety, and cardiovascular disease," *American Journal of Hypertension* 28, no. 11 (November 2015): 1295–302.
11. C. Smith, et al., "Primary care validation of a single-question alcohol screening test," Journal of General Internal Medicine 24, no. 7 (July 2009): 783–88.
12. Christopher & Dana Reeve Foundation, Paralysis Resource Guide. Accessed at christopherreeve.org/living-with-paralysis/free-resources-and-downloads/paralysis-resource-guide.

Chapter 2

1. The Resilience Project, theresilienceproject.com.au/about.
2. A. L. Boggiss, et al., "A systematic review of gratitude interventions: Effects on physical health and health behaviors," *Journal of Psychosomatic Research* 135 (August 2020): 110165.
   Brenda Nathan, *The One-Minute Gratitude Journal.* Self-Published, 2016.
3. Norman Doidge, *The Brain's Way of Healing: Remarkable Discoveries and Recoveries from the Frontiers of Neuroplasticity.* New York: Penguin Books, 2016.
4. A. Das, et al., "Beyond blindsight: properties of visual relearning in cortically blind fields," *Journal of Neuroscience* 34, no. 35 (August 2014): 11652–64.
5. Donald O. Hebb, The Organization of Behavior. New York: Wiley, 1949.
6. Peter G. Levine, *Stronger After Stroke: Your Roadmap to Recovery,* third ed. New York: Demos Health, 2018.

Chapter 4

1. Srinivasa N. Raja, et al., "The revised International Association for the Study of Pain definition of pain: concepts, challenges, and compromises," *Pain* 161, no. 9 (September 2020): 1976–82.
2. R. Baron, et al., "Neuropathic pain: Diagnosis, pathophysiological mechanisms, and treatment," *Lancet Neurology* 9, no. 8 (August 2010): 807–19.
   Gilron, et al., "Neuropathic pain: Principles of diagnosis and treatment," *Mayo Clin Proceedings* 90, no. 4 (April 2015): 532–45.
3. R. H. Dworkin, et al., "Recommendations for the pharmacological management of neuropathic pain: an overview and literature update," *Mayo Clinic Proceedings* 85, no. 3 (March 2010): S3–14.
4. US Food & Drug Administration, "FDA and Cannabis: Research and Drug Approval Process," October 2020. Accessed at www.fda.gov/news-events/public-health-focus/fda-and-cannabis-research-and-drug-approval-process.
5. E. Stockings, et al., "Cannabis and cannabinoids for the treatment of people with chronic noncancer pain conditions: a systematic review and meta-analysis of controlled and observational studies," Pain 159, no. 10 (October 2018): 1932–54.
6. S. M. Nugent, et al., "The Effects of Cannabis Among Adults With Chronic Pain and an Overview of General Harms: A Systematic Review," *Annals of Internal Medicine* 167, no. 5 (Sep 5 2017): 319–31.
7. D. I. Abrams, et al., "Cannabis in painful HIV-associated sensory neuropathy: a randomized placebo-controlled trial," Neurology 68, no. 7 (February 2007): 515–21.
   R. J. Ellis, et al., "Smoked medicinal cannabis for neuropathic pain in HIV: a randomized, crossover clinical trial," *Neuropsychopharmacology* 34, no. 3 (February 2009): 672–80.

B. Wilsey, et al., "A randomized, placebo-controlled, crossover trial of cannabis cigarettes in neuropathic pain," *Journal of Pain* 9, no. 6 (June 2008): 506–21.

8. M. S. Wallace, et al., "Efficacy of Inhaled Cannabis on Painful Diabetic Neuropathy," Journal of Pain 16, no. 7 (July 2015): 616–27.

B. Wilsey, et al., "Low-dose vaporized cannabis significantly improves neuropathic pain," *Journal of Pain* 14, no. 2 (February 2013): 136–48.

9. V. Challapalli, et al., "Systemic administration of local anesthetic agents to relieve neuropathic pain," *Cochrane Database of Systematic Reviews* 2005, no. 4 (October 2005): Cd003345.

E. Iacob, et al., "Tertiary Care Clinical Experience with Intravenous Lidocaine Infusions for the Treatment of Chronic Pain," *Pain Medicine* 19, no. 6 (June 2018): 1245–53.

10. D. M. Ehde, et al., "Cognitive-behavioral therapy for individuals with chronic pain: efficacy, innovations, and directions for research," *American Psychologist* 69, no. 2 (February/March 2014): 153–66.

11. Joseph Donnelly, et al., *Travell, Simons & Simons' Myofascial Pain and Dysfunction: The Trigger Point Manual*. Philadelphia: Wolters Kluwer, 2019.

12. Christopher & Dana Reeve Foundation, Paralysis Resource Guide, op cit.

T. Mokhtari et al., "Transcutaneous Electrical Nerve Stimulation in Relieving Neuropathic Pain: Basic Mechanisms and Clinical Applications," *Current Pain and Headache Reports* 24, no. 4 (February 2020): 14.

13. Steven Kirshblum and Denise Campagnolo, *Spinal Cord Medicine*. Philadelphia: Lippincott Williams & Wilkins, 2011.

J. J. Song, et al., "Present and potential use of spinal cord stimulation to control chronic pain," *Pain Physician* 17, no. 3 (May/June 2014): 235–46.

J. M. Meythaler, et al., "Intrathecal baclofen for spastic hypertonia from stroke," *Stroke* 32, no. 9 (September 2001): 2099–109.

14. J. De Andrés, et al., "Intrathecal Drug Delivery," *Methods in Molecular Biology* 2059 (August 2019): 75–108.

15. Y. H. Kuan and B. C. Shyu, "Nociceptive transmission and modulation via P2X receptors in central pain syndrome," *Molecular Brain* 9, no. 1 (May 2016): 58–67.

16. G. Z. Galafassi, et al., "Systematic Review: Neuromodulation for Medically Refractory Neuropathic Pain: spinal cord stimulation, deep brain stimulation, motor cortex stimulation and posterior insula stimulation," *World Neurosurgery* (November 2020): 246–60.

G. Mesaroli, et al., "Screening and diagnostic tools for complex regional pain syndrome: a systematic review," Pain (November 2020).

S. Yang and M. C. Chang, "Effect of Repetitive Transcranial Magnetic Stimulation on Pain Management: A Systematic Narrative Review," *Frontiers in Neurology* 11 (February 2020): 114.

Chapter 5

1. Brian Homewood, "Kipchoge's sub-two hour marathon like landing on the moon," *Reuters,* October 12, 2019.

2. Seth Gillihan, *Retrain Your Brain: Cognitive Behavioral Therapy in 7 Weeks, A Workbook for Managing Depression and Anxiety*. Berkeley: Althea Press, 2016.

Brian Tracy, *Goals! How to Get Everything You Want—Faster Than You Ever Thought Possible*. San Francisco: Berrett-Koehler Publishers, 2010.

Chapter 6

1. National Heart, Lung, and Blood Institute, "DASH Eating Plan." Accessed at www.nhlbi.nih.gov/health-topics/dash-eating-plan.
2. American Heart Association, "What is the Mediterranean Diet?" Accessed at heart.org/en/healthy-living/healthy-eating/eat-smart/nutrition-basics/mediterranean-diet.
3. Government of Canada, "A Consumer's Guide to the DRIs (Dietary Reference Intakes)." Accessed at canada.ca/en/health-canada/services/food-nutrition/healthy-eating/dietary-reference-intakes/consumer-guide-dris-dietary-reference-intakes.html.
4. Brain Injury Association, "Concussion Information Center." Accessed at biausa.org/public-affairs/media?search=%22concussion+information+center%22.
   Centers for Disease Control and Prevention, "Brain Injury Basics." Accessed at cdc.gov/headsup/basics/index.html.
5. R. Dong, et al., "Prevalence, Risk Factors, Outcomes, and Treatment of Obstructive Sleep Apnea in Patients with Cerebrovascular Disease: A Systematic Review," *Journal of Stroke & Cerebrovascular Diseases* 27, no. 6 (June 2018): 1471–80.
6. A. Lowe, et al., "Treatment of sleep disturbance following stroke and traumatic brain injury: a systematic review of conservative interventions," *Disability and Rehabilitation* (December 2020): 1–13.
7. S. Bogdanov, et al., "Sleep outcomes following sleep–hygiene–related interventions for individuals with traumatic brain injury: A systematic review," *Brain Injury* 31, no. 4 (2017): 422–33.
8. Lowe, *Disability and Rehabilitation*, op cit.
   J. Zhang, et al., "The effects of acupuncture versus sham/placebo acupuncture for insomnia: A systematic review and meta-analysis of randomized controlled trials," *Complement Therapies in Clinical Practice* 41 (November 2020): 1–13.

Chapter 7

1. E. S. Byers, "Relationship satisfaction and sexual satisfaction: a longitudinal study of individuals in long-term relationships," *Journal of Sex Research* 42, no. 2 (May 2005): 113–18.
   S. Litzinger and K. C. Gordon, "Exploring relationships among communication, sexual satisfaction, and marital satisfaction," *Journal of Sex &Marital Therapy* 31, no. 5 (October/December 2005): 409–24.
2. William H. Masters and Virginia E. Johnson, *Human Sexual Response*. New York: Ishi Press, 2010.
3. Steven Kirshblum and Denise Campagnolo, *Spinal Cord Medicine*. Philadelphia: Lippincott Williams & Wilkins, 2011.
4. Justin Lehmiller, "How Sexual Communication Differs From Nonsexual Communication," Kinsey Institute Research and Institute News, September 5, 2018.
   William R. Cupach and Jamie Comstock, "Satisfaction with Sexual Communication in Marriage: Links to Sexual Satisfaction and Dyadic Adjustment," *Journal of Social and Personal Relationships* 7, no. 2 (May 1990): 179–86.
   C. Quinn-Nilas, et al., "Validation of the Sexual Communication Self-Efficacy Scale," *Health Education & Behavior* 43, no. 2 (April 2016): 165–71.
5. L. Chen, et al., "Phosphodiesterase 5 inhibitors for the treatment of erectile dysfunction: A trade-off network meta-analysis," *European Urology* 68, no. 4 (October 2015): 674–80.

6. P. Oskui, et al., "Testosterone and the cardiovascular system: A comprehensive review of the clinical literature," *Journal of the American Heart Association* 2, no. 6 (November 2013): e000272.

R. Vigen, et al., "Association of testosterone therapy with mortality, myocardial infarction, and stroke in men with low testosterone levels," *JAMA* 310, no. 17 (November 2013): 1829–36.

J. L. Anderson, et al., "Impact of testosterone replacement therapy on myocardial infarction, stroke, and death in men with low testosterone concentrations in an integrated health care system," *American Journal of Cardiology* 117, no. 5 (March 2016): 794–9.

7. F. Courtois, et al., "Sexual function and autonomic dysreflexia in men with spinal cord injuries: how should we treat?" Spinal Cord 50, no. 12 (December 2012): 869–77.

A. Krassioukov, et al., "A systematic review of the management of autonomic dysreflexia after spinal cord injury," *Archives of Physical Medicine and Rehabilitation* 90, no. 4 (April 2009): 682–95.

Chapter 8

1. H. Beinfield and E. Korn, *Between Heaven and Earth: A Guide to Chinese Medicine.* New York: Ballantine Books, 1991.

2. T. C. Campbell, *The China Study: Startling Implications for Diet, Weight Loss, and Long-Term Health*. Dallas: BenBella Books, 2006.

3. T. C. Campbell and T. M. Campbell II, *The China Study: The Most Comprehensive Study of Nutrition Ever Conducted and the Startling Implications for Diet, Weight Loss, and Long-Term Health,* revised and expanded edition. Dallas: BenBella Books, 2016.

4. D. Mohan, et al., "Associations of fish consumption with risk of cardiovascular disease and mortality among individuals with or without vascular disease from 58 countries," *JAMA Internal Medicine* (March 2021): e210036.

H. Choi, et al., "Omega-3 fatty acids supplementation on major cardiovascular outcomes: An umbrella review of meta-analyses of observational studies and randomized controlled trials," *European Review for Medical and Pharmacological Sciences* 25, no. 4 (February 2021): 2079–92.

5. D. L. Bhatt, et al., "Cardiovascular risk reduction with icosapent ethyl for hypertriglyceridemia," *New England Journal of Medicine* 380, no. 1 (January 2019): 11–22.

6. J. M. Brown and S. L. Hazen, "Targeting of microbe-derived metabolites to improve human health: The next frontier for drug discovery," *Journal of Biological Chemistry* 292, no. 21 (May 2017): 8560–68.

7. National Center for Complementary and Integrative Health, "Complementary, Alternative, or Integrative Health: What's In a Name?" Accessed at nccih.nih.gov/health/complementary-alternative-or-integrative-health-whats-in-a-name.

8. J. A. Astin, et al., "A review of the incorporation of complementary and alternative medicine by mainstream physicians," *Archives of Internal Medicine* 158, no. 21 (November 1998): 2303–10.

9. L. Johnston, "Alternative, complementary, energy-based medicine for spinal cord injury," *Acta Neurochirugica Supplement* 93 (2005): 155–58.

10. M. V. Madsen, et al., "Acupuncture treatment for pain: systematic review of randomised clinical trials with acupuncture, placebo acupuncture, and no acupuncture groups," *BMJ* 338 (January 2009): a3115.

11. M. Moayedi and K. D. Davis, "Theories of pain: from specificity to gate control," *Journal of Neurophysiology* 109, no. 1 (January 2013): 5–12.

12. O. Dupuy, et al., "An Evidence-Based Approach for Choosing Post-exercise Recovery Techniques to Reduce Markers of Muscle Damage, Soreness, Fatigue, and Inflammation: A Systematic Review With Meta-Analysis," *Frontiers in Physiology* 9 (April 2018): 403.

13. C. A. Brown and A. K. Jones, "Psychobiological correlates of improved mental health in patients with musculoskeletal pain after a mindfulness-based pain management program," *Clinical Journal of Pain* 29, no. 3 (March 2013): 233–44.

    M. Goyal, et al., "Meditation programs for psychological stress and well-being: a systematic review and meta-analysis," *JAMA Internal Medicine* 174, no. 3 (March 2014): 357–68.

    E. L. Khoo, et al., "Comparative evaluation of group-based mindfulness-based stress reduction and cognitive behavioural therapy for the treatment and management of chronic pain: A systematic review and network meta-analysis," *Evidence-Based Mental Health* 22, no. 1 (February 2019): 26–35.

14. Brown and Jones, *Clinical Journal of Pain,* op cit.

15. Department of Family Medicine and Community Health, "Mindfulness Resources." Accessed at: fammed.wisc.edu/mindfulness/resources.

16. Dan Hurley, "Breathing In vs. Spacing Out," *The New York Times Magazine,* January 14, 2014.

    M. V. Rainforth, et al., "Stress reduction programs in patients with elevated blood pressure: a systematic review and meta-analysis," *Current Hypertension Reports* 9, no. 6 (December 2007): 520–28.

    J. O. Younge, et al., "Mind-body practices for patients with cardiac disease: a systematic review and meta-analysis," *European Journal of Preventive Cardiology* 22, no. 11 (November 2015): 1385–98.

17. Younge, *European Journal of Preventive Cardiology* 2, op cit.

    E. C. Gathright, et al., "The impact of transcendental meditation on depressive symptoms and blood pressure in adults with cardiovascular disease: A systematic review and meta-analysis," *Complementary Therapies in Medicine* 46 (October 2019): 172–79.

18. Department of Family Medicine and Community Health, "Meditation for Health & Happiness: Overview for Clinicians." Accessed at fammed.wisc.edu/integrative/resources/modules/meditation.

19. A. Qaseem, et al., "Noninvasive Treatments for Acute, Subacute, and Chronic Low Back Pain: A Clinical Practice Guideline From the American College of Physicians," *Annals of Internal Medicine* 166, no. 7 (April 2017): 514–30.

    C. A. Smith, et al., "Relaxation techniques for pain management in labour," Cochrane *Database of Systematic Reviews* 3, no. 3 (March 2018): Cd009514 1–77.

20. S. Telles, et al., "Yoga: Can It Be Integrated with Treatment of Neuropathic Pain," *Integrative Medicine International* 4, no. 1–2 (August 2017): 69–84.

21. Matthew Sanford, *Waking: A Memoir of Trauma and Transcendence.* Emmaus, PA: Rodale Publishing, 2008.

22. B. K. S. Iyengar, *Light on Yoga: The Bible of Modern Yoga.* New York: Schocken Books, 1979.

23. R. L. Nahin et al. "Expenditures on Complementary Health Approaches: United States, 2012," *National Health Statistics Report,* no. 95 (Jun 22 2016): 1–11.

Chapter 9

1. T. Sugimura, et al., "Chronic suprapubic catheterization in the management of patients with spinal cord injuries: Analysis of upper and lower urinary tract complications," *BJU International* 101, no. 11 (June 2008): 1396–1400.

2. Q. Q. Gong, et al., "Meta-analysis of randomized controlled trials using botulinum toxin a at different dosages for urinary incontinence in patients with overactive bladder," *Frontiers in Pharmacology* 10 (January 2020): 1618.

Chapter 11

1. P. Jha, et al., "21st-century hazards of smoking and benefits of cessation in the United States," *New England Journal of Medicine* 368, no. 4 (January 2013): 341–50.

Chapter 13

1. Kirshblum and Campagnolo, *Spinal Cord Medicine,* op cit.

Chapter 14

1. C. A. Angeli, et al., "Recovery of Over-Ground Walking after Chronic Motor Complete Spinal Cord Injury," *New England Journal of Medicine* 379, no. 13 (September 2018): 1244–50.
2. Kirshblum and Campagnolo, *Spinal Cord Medicine,* op cit.
3. H. M. Lau, et al., "The effectiveness of thoracic manipulation on patients with chronic mechanical neck pain—a randomized controlled trial," *Manual Therapy* 16, no. 2 (April 2011): 141–47.
4. F. M. Ivey, et al., "Strength Training for Skeletal Muscle Endurance after Stroke," *Journal of Stroke & Cerebrovascular Diseases* 26, no. 4 (April 2017): 787–94.
   M. S. Fragala, et al., "Muscle quality index improves with resistance exercise training in older adults," *Experimental Gerontology* 53 (May 2014): 1–6.
5. K. A. Stockton, et al., "Effect of vitamin D supplementation on muscle strength: a systematic review and meta-analysis," *Osteoporosis International* 22, no. 3 (March 2011): 859–71.

Chapter 19

1. S. Harkema, et al., "Effect of epidural stimulation of the lumbosacral spinal cord on voluntary movement, standing, and assisted stepping after motor complete paraplegia: a case study," *Lancet* 377, no. 9781 (June 2011): 1938–47.
2. N. Cho, et al., "Neurorestorative interventions involving bioelectronic implants after spinal cord injury," *Bioelectronic Medicine* 5 (July 2019): 10–29.
   F. B. Wagner, et al., "Targeted neurotechnology restores walking in humans with spinal cord injury," *Nature* 563, no. 7729 (November 2018): 65–71.
   E. Formento, et al., "Electrical spinal cord stimulation must preserve proprioception to enable locomotion in humans with spinal cord injury," *Nature Neuroscience* 21, no. 12 (December 2018): 1728–41.
3. Cho, *Bioelectronic Medicine,* op cit.
4. Wagner, *Nature,* op cit.
5. Liza V. McHugh, et al., "Feasibility and utility of transcutaneous spinal cord stimulation combined with walking-based therapy for people with motor incomplete spinal cord injury," *Spinal Cord Series and Cases* 6, no. 1 (November 2020): 104.
6. Cho, *Bioelectronic Medicine,* op cit.
   Wagner, *Nature,* op cit.

7. Cho, *Bioelectronic Medicine,* op cit.
8. R. Yawn, et al., "Cochlear implantation: a biomechanical prosthesis for hearing loss," *F1000Prime Reports* 7 (April 2015): 45.
9. Yawn, *F1000Prime Reports,* op cit.
10. F. Herpich, et al., "Boosting Learning Efficacy with Noninvasive Brain Stimulation in Intact and Brain-Damaged Humans," *Journal of Neuroscience* 39, no. 28 (July 2019): 5551–61.
11. S. S. Shin, et al., "Neurostimulation for traumatic brain injury," *Journal of Neurosurgery* 121, no. 5 (November 2014): 1219–31.
    T. Tazoe and M. A. Perez, "Effects of repetitive transcranial magnetic stimulation on recovery of function after spinal cord injury," *Archives of Physical Medicine and Rehabilitation* 96, no. 4 (April 2015): S145–55.
12. A. L. Benabid, et al., "An exoskeleton controlled by an epidural wireless brain-machine interface in a tetraplegic patient: a proof-of-concept demonstration," *Lancet Neurology* 18, no. 12 (December 2019): 1112–22.
13. W. A. El-Kheir, et al., "Autologous bone marrow-derived cell therapy combined with physical therapy induces functional improvement in chronic spinal cord injury patients," *Cell Transplantation* 23, no. 6 (April 2014): 729–45.
14. El-Kheir, *Cell Transplantation,* op cit.
15. M. Kawabori, et al., "Clinical Trials of Stem Cell Therapy for Cerebral Ischemic Stroke," *International Journal of Molecular Sciences* 21, no. 19 (October 2020): 7380.
16. Kawabori, *International Journal of Molecular Sciences,* op cit.
17. G. Schepici, et al., "Traumatic Brain Injury and Stem Cells: An Overview of Clinical Trials, the Current Treatments and Future Therapeutic Approaches," Medicina (Kaunas, Lithuania) 56, no. 3 (March 2020): 1–14, 137.
18. S. Wang, et al., "Umbilical cord mesenchymal stem cell transplantation significantly improves neurological function in patients with sequelae of traumatic brain injury," *Brain Research* 1532 (September 2013): 76–84.
19. H. Katoh, et al., "Regeneration of Spinal Cord Connectivity Through Stem Cell Transplantation and Biomaterial Scaffolds," *Frontiers in Cellular Neuroscience* 13 (June 2019): 248.
20. F. Ghin, et al., "The effects of high-frequency transcranial random noise stimulation (hf-tRNS) on global motion processing: An equivalent noise approach," *Brain Stimulation* 11, no. 6 (November/December 2018): 1263–75.
21. Herpich, *Journal of Neuroscience,* op cit.
22. M. L. Ettenhofer, et al., "Neurocognitive Driving Rehabilitation in Virtual Environments (NeuroDRIVE): A pilot clinical trial for chronic traumatic brain injury," *NeuroRehabilitation* 44, no. 4 (July 2019): 531–44.
    M. G. Maggio, et al., "The Growing Use of Virtual Reality in Cognitive Rehabilitation: Fact, Fake or Vision? A Scoping Review," *Journal of the National Medical Association* 111, no. 4 (August 2019): 457–63.
    E. B. Larson, et al., "Tolerance of a virtual reality intervention for attention remediation in persons with severe TBI," *Brain Injury* 25, no. 3 (2011): 274–81.
    R. J. Matheis, et al., "Is learning and memory different in a virtual environment?" *Clinical Neuropsychologist* 21, no. 1 (January 2007): 146–61.
    A. Miguel-Rubio, et al., "Is Virtual Reality Effective for Balance Recovery in Patients with Spinal Cord Injury? A Systematic Review and Meta-Analysis," *Journal of Clinical Medicine* 9, no. 9 (September 2020).
    A. De Miguel-Rubio, et al., "Virtual Reality Systems for Upper Limb Motor Function Recovery in Patients With Spinal Cord Injury: Systematic Review and

Meta-Analysis," *JMIR Mhealth and Uhealth* 8, no. 12 (December 2020): e22537.

D. Charles, et al., "Virtual Reality Design for Stroke Rehabilitation," Advances in Experimental Medicine and Biology 1235 (2020): 53–87.

R. Cassani, et al., "Virtual reality and non-invasive brain stimulation for rehabilitation applications: a systematic review," *Journal of NeuroEngineering and Rehabilitation* 17, no. 1 (October 2020): 1–16, 147.

23. M. G. Maggio, et al., "Cognitive rehabilitation in patients with traumatic brain injury: A narrative review on the emerging use of virtual reality," *Journal of Clinical Neuroscience* 61 (March 2019): 1–4.

24. J. W. Grau, et al., "Learning to promote recovery after spinal cord injury," *Experimental Neurology* 330 (August 2020): 1–20, 113334.

25. D. Di Raimondo, et al., "Role of Regular Physical Activity in Neuroprotection against Acute Ischemia," *International Journal of Molecular Sciences* 21, no. 23 (November 2020): 1–30, 9086.

26. H. Quan, et al., "Exercise, redox system and neurodegenerative diseases," *Biochimica et Biophysica Acta – Molecular Basis of Disease* 1866, no. 10 (October 2020): 165778.

27. M. T. Joy and S. T. Carmichael, "Encouraging an excitable brain state: mechanisms of brain repair in stroke," *Nature Reviews Neuroscience* 22, no. 1 (January 2021): 38–53.

28. D. A. Tran, et al., "Combining Dopaminergic Facilitation with Robot-Assisted Upper Limb Therapy in Stroke Survivors: A Focused Review," *American Journal of Physical Medicine & Rehabilitation* 95, no. 6 (June 2016): 459–74.

K. Molina-Luna, et al., "Dopamine in motor cortex is necessary for skill learning and synaptic plasticity," *PLoS One* 4, no. 9 (September 2009): e7082.

29. A. M. Bakheit, "Drug treatment of poststroke aphasia," *Expert Review of Neurotherapeutics* 4, no. 2 (March 2004): 211–17.

S. E. Nadeau, et al., "Donepezil as an adjuvant to constraint-induced therapy for upper-limb dysfunction after stroke: an exploratory randomized clinical trial," *Journal of Rehabilitation Research & Development* 41, no. 4 (July 2004): 525–34.

30. G. Batsikadze et al., "Effect of serotonin on paired associative stimulation-induced plasticity in the human motor cortex," *Neuropsychopharmacology* 38, no. 11 (October 2013): 2260–67.

C. B. Pinto, et al., "SSRI and Motor Recovery in Stroke: Reestablishment of Inhibitory Neural Network Tonus," *Frontiers in Neuroscience* 11 (November 2017): 637.

31. Y. Tang, et al., "P2X receptors and acupuncture analgesia," *Brain Research Bulletin* 151 (September 2019): 144–52.

J. Sawynok, "Adenosine receptor targets for pain," *Neuroscience* 338 (December 2016): 1–18.

32. M. Koszewicz, et al., "Dysbiosis is one of the risk factor for stroke and cognitive impairment and potential target for treatment," *Pharmacological Research* (November 2020): 105277.

33. G. C. Román, et al., "Mediterranean diet: The role of long-chain ω-3 fatty acids in fish; polyphenols in fruits, vegetables, cereals, coffee, tea, cacao and wine; probiotics and vitamins in prevention of stroke, age-related cognitive decline, and Alzheimer disease," *Revue Neurologique* (Paris) 175, no. 10 (December 2019): 724–41.

34. M. W. Rice, et al., "Gut Microbiota as a Therapeutic Target to Ameliorate the Biochemical, Neuroanatomical, and Behavioral Effects of Traumatic Brain Injuries," *Frontiers in Neurology* 10 (August 2019): 875.

Image Credits

Figure 1 © Maya E. Habecker

Figures 2A © Henry Vandyke Carter, Wikimedia Commons; B, C © Ralf Stephan, Wikimedia Commons

Figures 3, 4, 5 © Bradford C. Berk and Shehanaz Ellika

Figure 6 © David Goldstein, open access

Figures 7A © Deutsche Fotothek, Wikimedia Commons; B © Susanne Pallo, URMC Communications

Figure 8 © Scott Medical

Figures 9, 10, 22, 32, 33, 38, Table 1 © Bradford C. Berk

Figure 11 © Farcaster, Wikimedia Commons

Figure 12 © Yeza, Wikimedia Commons

Figures 13A © Blausen.com; B © Mconnell, Wikimedia Commons

Figures 14, 16, 17, 18A, B adapted by Michal Shaposhnikov and Bradford C. Berk

Figure 15 public domain, Wikimedia Commons

Figures 19A, B © BruceBlaus, Wikimedia Commons

Figure 20 © Ucomfor, adapted by Michal Shaposhnikov and Bradford C. Berk

Figure 21 © William Crochot, Wikimedia Commons

Figures 23, 24 Wikipedia Commons

Figure 25 © Nanoxyde, Wikimedia Commons

Figure 26 © Neuromotion Physiotherapy

Figure 27 © Christopher & Dana Reeve Foundation

Figures 28A, B © Hocoma

Figures 29A, B © ReWalk

Figure 30 © Nick Yudin, Wikimedia Commons, adapted by Michal Shaposhnikov and Bradford C. Berk

Figure 31 © Open Access Resources

Figure 34 © Reharo Corporation

Figure 35 © EazyHold, Mellin Works, LLC

Figure 36 © Dining with Dignity

Figure 37 © GF Health Products, Inc.

Table 2 adapted by Bradford C. Berk from C. T. January, L. S. Wann, H. Calkins, L. Y. Chen, et al

Table 3 adapted by Bradford C. Berk from Steven Kirshblum and Denise Campagnolo

Index

NOTE: Page numbers in *italics* indicate a graphic or photograph.

chronic neurogenic bladder, 132, 143
and sexual healing, 110
spasm prevention and defense, 138
toileting aids, 213
See also digestive tract health
bowel management outside the home, 153
bowel program, 148, 150, 154
bradycardia, 162
brain
overview, *10*, 11–12, *13*
cerebrum and cerebellum, *10*, 12
depression and activation procedures,
29–30
and functional MRI, 119
proprioception, 208
and sexual arousal, 108–109
stroke damage, *14*
TBI damage, *15*
Brain Injury Association of America (BIAA),
97
brain-computer interface (BCI), 199, 256
brain-derived neurotrophic factor (BDNF),
264
breathing problems after ANI, 167
breathing, strengthening your, 169–171
Broca's area of the brain, *10*, 12
bronchospasm, 168
bus tours, 237

CAD (atherosclerosis in the coronary arteries), 157
calcium score, 161
calendar of daily events, 89
Calimeris, Dorothy, 95
CAM (complementary and alternative medicine), 118–119, 125–126, 127
Campbell, T. Colin, 118
Campbell, Thomas M., 118
canes, 208
cannabidiol (CBD), 73–74
cannabis and cannabinoids, 72–74
capsaicin, 75
cardiac catherization and angiogram, 161
cardiovascular disease (CVD)
overview, 156, 157
and cholesterol, 158–159
purified fish oil vs., 118
risk factors, 156–157
and smoking, 158
and testosterone level, 112–113

and type 2 diabetes, 157–158
cardiovascular system, 156, *156*
caregivers, 35, 41, 62
carpal tunnel syndrome (CTS), 188
carpets as a trip hazard, 220
catastrophic thinking, 41
CBD (cannabidiol), 73–74
CBT (cognitive behavioral therapy)
overview, 37–38, 77
for anxiety, 31
for chronic stress and anxiety, 99
combining with support groups, 34
for depression, 28
exposure therapy with, 32
for grief treatment, 26–27
including in treatment plan, 22–23
for PTSD, 32
Celebrex (celecoxib), 29
Centers for Disease Control and Prevention
(CDC), 97
central nervous system
and cerebrum of the brain, 12
damage and muscle atrophy, 183
pain from damage to, 70, 83, 183
Tootsie Roll pop analogy, 11
Central Pain Syndrome, 82–83
central pattern generators (CPGs), 252
cerebral cortex, *10*, 12
cerebrum and cerebellum of the brain, *10*,
12
certified home health aide, 56
CHA2DS2-VASc score, 163
checking in at airports, 233–234
China. *See* traditional Chinese medicine
China Study, The (Campbell and Campbell),
118
Chinese diet, 118, 126, 271
cholesterol and CVD, 158–159
chronic depression, 25–26
chronic pain, 69
chronic traumatic encephalopathy (CTE),
2
Churchill, Winston, 92
clinical trials, 250, 266–267
clothing aids, 214
cognitive behavioral therapy. *See* CBT
collapsed lung, 166, 168–169
colonoscopy, 148
communication with your partner about
intimacy, 106–108, 116

community
  getting around in your wheelchair, 206–207
  quitting smoking, 99
  resources specific to your, 51–52, 91
  wellness program, 96
  See also thriving in your community
compensation and neuroplasticity, 44
complementary and alternative medicine
  (CAM), 118–119, 125–126, 127
complementary medicine therapies for
  PTSD, 32
Complete Anti-Inflammatory Diet for Beginners
  (Calimeris), 95
complex regional pain syndrome (CRPS),
  49, 79, 83–84, 121, 189, 255, 274
complicated grief, 26–27
computers, 197
condom catheter, 135, *135*
consciousness, state of, 43–44
constipation, 144–145, 148, 150, 151, 154
*Consumer's Guide to the DRIs (Dietary Refer-
  ence Intakes)* (Health Canada), 96
continuing-care model of substance abuse
  with a chronic disease, 33, 34
continuity of care at rehab facility, 53
continuous positive airway pressure (CPAP),
  100
corpus callosum of the brain, *10*, 12
coughing to dislodge mucus plugs, 171–172
CPAP (continuous positive airway pressure),
  100, 169
CPAP (continuous-positive airway pressure),
  169
CPGs (central pattern generators), 252
cranberry juice for UTIs, 142
Credé's maneuver, 134
CRPS (complex regional pain syndrome),
  49, 79, 83–84, 121, 189, 255, 274
cruises, 239
crutches, 208
cryotherapy, 78
CT (computerized tomography) calcium
  score, 161
CTE (chronic traumatic encephalopathy), 2
Cuylenburg, Hugh van, 39–43
CVD. *See* cardiovascular disease (CVD)

D-mannose, 140
DASH (Dietary Approaches to Stop Hypertension), 94–95

debridement of pressure ulcers, 179
denial with ANI grieving process, 24–25
dental hygiene, 140–141
Department of Veterans Affairs, 224
Department of Vocational Rehabilitation,
  state, 224
depression
  overview, 2
  brain activation therapy, 29–30
  conditions that mimic depression, 27
  and exercise, 30
  in grieving process, 25–26
  overcoming, 7
  treatment for, 27–30
  See also CBT
devices. *See* adaptive devices, tools, and more
diagnoses
  anxiety, 31
  of anxiety disorders, 31
  complicated grief, 26
  depression, 27
  fecal incontinence, 152
  heart disease, 160–161
  post-operative spine degeneration, 191
  SIRS, 164
diclofenac (Flector) patch, 75
diet
  overview, 94
  and bowel function, 149
  Chinese diet, 118, 126, 271
  and fecal incontinence, 152
  and pressure ulcer prevention, 178
  protein, for sarcopenia recovery, 192
dietary counseling, 95–96
digestive tract health, 144–154
  overview, 154
  anatomy of the GI tract, 144–145, *145*
  bowel management outside the home, 153
  fecal incontinence, 152–153
  importance of food, 144
  neurogenic bowel, 147–151
  swallowing and dysphagia, 145–147
  See also bowel and bladder function
Dining with Dignity fork, 215, *215*
Disability and Business Technical Assistance
  Centers, 227
disability insurance, 36, 243–244
discharge planner, 51, 52, 56
discharge, plans for, 51–63
  assistive devices, 58

external pressure ulcers, 175
extubation, 168
eyesight recovery, 45, *45*

Fair Employment Practice Agency (FEPA), 227
fall prevention, 210–211
family as support system, 35–36, 93
fatigue, 140
fecal incontinence, 145, 152–153, 154
fertility issues, 114–115, 116
FES (functional electrical stimulation), 181, 183, *184*
fiber, 149
fibrosis, 167
finances
  finding funds for services, 56
  insurance plans, 58–62, *59*, 60, 61, 62
  paying for your adaptive devices, 217–218
  paying for your rehabilitation facility, 90–92
  paying for your trip, 231
  and wheelchair purchase, 201, 202, 203
financial counseling, 36
five elements (wood, water, fire, earth, and metal), 120
Flector (diclofenac) patch, 75
flexor tendonitis, lateral and medial, 188–189
flu vaccinations, 171
fluid intake, 141, 149
foam beds, 200
focus as a mental tool, 40, 41–42
Foley catheter, 133, *133*, 137
Food and Drug Administration (FDA), 73–74, 82
foundations that support people with disabilities, 91
four-wheel walker, 209, *209*
friction damage to skin, 176
friends
  post-trauma communion with, 241–242
  as support system, 35–36, 93
front-wheeled walker, 208–209, *209*
frontal lobe of the brain, *10*, 11–12
frozen shoulder, muscle overuse injury, 187–188
functional electrical stimulation (FES), 181, 183, *184*
functional recovery, 181

Funding Resources Guide, 217
Fung, Jason, 95
future therapies, 249–267
  overview, 267
  clinical trials, 250, 266–267
  devices, 249, 250–262
  integrative medicine, 250, 265–266
  neuroplasticity enhanced by drugs and devices, 249–250, 262–265
  regenerative medicine, 250, 258–261

gastrointestinal system, 143, 144–145, *145*
GI tract, 144–145, *145*
Glasgow Coma Scale (GCS), 43–44
Goldstein, David, 11–12
gratitude and gratitude journal, 41, 50
Greger, Michael, 95
grief, 24, 26–27, 37
grieving process, 21–23, 24–26
grooming aids, 213–214
gut microbiome, 142

HDL (high-density lipoprotein), 158–159
health care team
  choosing your wheelchair, 202
  identifying goals and consulting with your team, 87
  multidisciplinary team, 38
  as part of your support system, 36–37
  prescription for your vehicle eliminates sales tax, 225
  during rehabilitation, 55–56
  talking with you and your loved ones, 31
  treating type 2 diabetes, 158
  on using a standard frame, 212
hearing sensory devices, 254
heart health, 155–165
  overview, 164–165
  diagnosis and evaluation of heart disease, 160–161
  need for disease prevention measures, 155
  See also cardiovascular disease
heat stroke, 162
Hebbian theory, 45
hemorrhagic stroke, *14*
herbs and supplements, 125–126, 127
heterotopic ossification, 191
high-density lipoprotein (HDL), 158–159
hippocampus of the brain, *10*, 12
Hocoma Lokomat robot, 186, *186*

home accessibility and wheelchair choice, 206
home renovations, 91
home, rehabilitation at, 53–54, 55
hospital-aquired pneumonia, 167
How Not to Diet (Greger), 95
Hoyer lift, 216, *216*
Human Sexual Response (Masters and Johnson), 108
hydrotherapy, 78
hygiene aids, 213–214
hypertension, 101, 112, 159
hypertrophy, 182

IDD (intrathecal drug delivery), 81, *82*
immobility and muscle atrophy, 182
incentive spirometer for lung health, 167, *170*, 170–171
incontinence, 132, 145, 152–153, 154
insurance plans, 58–62, *59*, 60, 61, 62
integrative medicine, 117–119, 126, 250, 265–266
International Association for the Study of Pain, 67
intestinal motility, 150
intimacy. *See* sexual healing
intrathecal drug delivery (IDD) "pain pump," 81, *82*
invasive pain therapies, 81–82
ischemic stroke, *14*, 157

Johnson, Virginia E., 108
joint motion, heterotopic ossification vs., 191
journal
   of daily events, 89
   of diet, 149
   gratitude journal, 41, 50
   of interactions with insurer, 90
   list of devices of interest, 198

KAFO (knee-ankle-foot orthosis), 207
Kessler Rehabilitation Center, New Jersey, 39, 53, 54
kidney stones, 136
kidneys, *131*, 132, 134, 136, 140
Kipchoge, Eliud, 88
kitchen accessibility, 222
knee braces, 208
knee replacement story, 2

knee-ankle-foot orthosis (KAFO), 207
Kübler-Ross model of grieving, 24–26

lateral and medial epicondylitis, 188–189
laxatives, 151
LDL (low-density lipoprotein), 158–159
learning and neuroplasticity, 44
Levine, Peter G., 46–47
Li, Jianan, 117
libido decrease, 114, 116
lidocaine (Lidoderm) patch, 75
lidocaine infusion, 75
life planner, 36
lifestyle = wellness, 94–101
   overview, 94, 101
   alcohol and ANI, *96*
   consulting with a nutritionist, 95–96
   DASH diet and Mediterranean diet, 94–95
   effect of weight on recovery, 98
   harmful effects of smoking, 98–99
   sleep, 100–101
   smoking vs., 98–99
   stress, 99
   supplements, 96–97
Lokomat treadmill, 185, *185*
low-density lipoprotein (LDL), 158–159
lung health, 166–172
   overview, 166, 172
   lung problems, 166–169
   lung secretions and mucus, 171–172
   treatments to improve lung health, 169–171

magical thinking, 25
magnesium citrate, 151
management of dysphagia, 147
mantras, 26–27
manual wheelchairs, *202*, 203
MAS (mobile arm support), 214
Masako maneuver while swallowing, 147
massage therapist, 122
massage therapy, 79, 80
massed practice for neurorehabilitation, 46–48
Masters, William H., 108
mattress materials, 200–201
mechanical lung problems, 166
Medicaid coverage, 36, 60
medical emergencies while traveling, 239–240

nervous system; peripheral nervous system

SSRIs (selective serotonin reuptake inhibitors), 28–29, 31, 32, 99

standard walker, 208, *209*

standing and exercise, for intestinal motility, 150

standing frames, 150, 212

state building codes for accessibility, 220–221

static flotation beds, 200–201

stem cells and stem cell therapy, 258–261

stimulant laxatives, 151

stimulation protocols for devices, 252

stress, 99, 140

stroke patients
  overview, 14, *14*
  aphasia from, 86
  and atrial fibrillation, 163
  and Central Pain Syndrome, 83–84
  DASH diet applicable to, 95
  dysphagia risk factors, 146
  exosuits designed for, 210
  gentle exercise program for, 97–98
  and heart disease, 157
  heart health problems, 163
  and neurogenic bladder, 132
  NSAIDs for, 29
  prescribing exercise for, 30
  sexual function after, 109
  sleep disturbances associated with, 100
  survivor's neuroplasticity, 44
  thromboembolic stroke risk predictor, 163, *163*
  See also ANI

Strong Memorial Hospital, Rochester, 39, 61, 69

Stronger After Stroke (Levine), 46–47

substance abuse, 33–34

Supplemental Security Income (SSI), 244

supplements, 96–97

supplements and herbs, 125–126, 127

support groups
  for aphasia, 86
  learning solutions of your peers, 242
  for loved ones of ANI survivors, 36
  Push Men, 268
  for substance abuse victims, 34

support surfaces and pressure ulcers, 177–178

support system (psychosocial network), 35–37, 93

suppositories for bowel movements, 151

suprapubic tube (SPT) catheter, 136, *136*, 137

surgery
  for fecal incontinence, 153
  for pressure ulcer debridement, 179–180
  surgical implants for men, 113

suspension systems, 185, *185*

swallowing and dysphagia, 145–147

swallowing study, 146–147, 154

sympathetic nervous system (SNS), 77

systemic inflammatory response syndrome (SIRS), 164

tai chi, 125

task-specific model for neurorehabilitation, 46–47

TBI (traumatic brain injury) patients
  overview, 2, 11, 15, *15*
  aphasia from, 86
  balance challenges, 86
  and Central Pain Syndrome, 83–84
  dysphagia risk factors, 146
  heart health problems, 164
  pituitary hormone insufficiency, 115
  sexual function after, 109
  and SIRS, 164
  sleep disturbances associated with, 100
  and SSRI treatment, 29

TCAs (tricyclic antidepressants), 28, 29

TCM (traditional Chinese medicine)
  overview, 117–119, 120
  acupuncture, 120–121, *121*
  Chinese diet, 118, 126, 271
  focus on mechanisms that regulate function, 119
  massage, 121–122
  philosophy of, 119–120
  and supplements, 126
  therapies for ANI, 120–124

temperature regulation, 162

temperature sensory devices, 254–255

temporal lobe of the brain, *10*, 11–12

TENS (transcutaneous electrical nerve stimulation), 80–81, *81*, 83

tension rings, 113

tetrahydrocannabinol (THC), 73, 74

THC (tetrahydrocannabinol), 73, 74

thermotherapy, 78

thinking, 43

thriving in your community, 241–248

About the Authors

BRADFORD C. BERK, MD, PhD, is a board-certified cardiologist and a Distinguished University Professor in Medicine, Neurology, Pathology, and Pharmacology & Physiology. Currently, he is the director of the University of Rochester Neurorestoration Institute (URNI).

Dr. Berk was recruited to URMC in 1998 as chief of the Cardiology Division. Prior to his recruitment to Rochester, he served on the faculties of Harvard Medical School, Emory University, and the University of Washington. He founded URMC's Aab Cardiovascular Research Institute, which rapidly became one of the nation's top ten most highly funded cardiovascular research programs. Dr. Berk served as Chairman of Medicine from 2001 until 2006. In 2006, Dr. Berk became CEO of URMC and Senior Vice President of Health Sciences at the University of Rochester.

In 2015, Dr. Berk stepped down as CEO and became the founding director of the URNI. The mission of the URNI is to bring the highest-quality multidisciplinary care and most innovative approaches to restore function in individuals who have suffered damage to their brain, spinal cord, and peripheral nerves.

His research has focused on understanding the molecular mechanisms of cardiovascular disease; specifically, the roles of oxidative stress and inflammation in the development and progression of disease. Recently, he has been studying the role of inflammation in acute and chronic spinal cord injury. He also is one of the founding members of NeuroCuresNY, the first large-scale clinical research platform that will use an upper-limb robot to investigate the effects of drugs to improve stroke recovery.

PRINCE ALBERT PUBLIC LIBRARY
31234900118439
Getting your brain and body back : every

He is on the editorial boards of *Circulation*, *Circulation Research*, and the *Journal of Clinical Investigation*, and he has published more than three hundred articles, chapters, and books.

Dr. Berk serves on the Empire State Stem Cell Board. He was a member of the National Heart Lung and Blood Institute (NHLBI) Advisory Council that functions as the advisory group to the director of NHLBI. He has served as chairman of the National Institutes of Health Vascular Biology study section, on the American Heart Association Scientific Research Council, and numerous international scientific review committees. He was also president of the North American Vascular Biology Organization. Dr. Berk is an elected member of the Association of American Physicians and the American Society of Clinical Investigation.

Dr. Berk is married to Dr. Coral Surgeon. He has three grown children (who have three terrific spouses) and seven grandchildren. He is an avid skier and cyclist and loves to travel. He collects wines, art, and good times with family and friends. He lives and works in Rochester, New York.

drbradberk.com | ⓘ drbradberk

MARTHA WATSON MURPHY is an award-winning author who has written, co-written, edited, or developed more than thirty books. Her areas of interest include health; food and the people who bring it to us; life in out-of-the-way places; how-to; memoir; business; and our relationship with dogs.